Nursing At Night
A Professional Approach

Nursing At Night
A Professional Approach

Edited by
Richard McMahon

SCUTARI PRESS
London

© Scutari Press 1992

A division of Scutari Projects, the publishing company of the Royal College of Nursing.

First published 1992

British Library Cataloguing in Publication Data
Nursing at night: a professional approach.
  I. McMahon, Richard
  610.73

  ISBN 1–871364–72–8

Phototypeset by Intype, London
Printed and bound in Great Britain by Unwin Brothers Ltd.,
The Gresham Press, Old Woking, Surrey, GU22 9LH.

Contents

Contributors

Joanne Blake, RGN, Dip N, Cert Ed, RNT
Formerly Nurse Teacher, Powys Health Authority

Anne Cawthorn, RGN, OND, Dip N(Lond), Cert Ed, RNT
Nurse Tutor, Stockport, Tameside and Glossop College of Nursing

S. José Closs, BSc(Hons) RGN, M Phil
Research Associate, Nursing Research Unit, University of Edinburgh

Anne Louise De Raeve, BA, RGN
Macmillan Lecturer in Nursing Ethics, Centre for Philosophy and Health Care, University College of Swansea

Simon Folkard, BSc, PhD, DSc, C Psychol, FBPsS
Senior Scientist, MRC/ESRC Social and Applied Psychology Unit, University of Sheffield

Fiona Hicks, BSc(Hons), DMS, RGN
Clinical Nurse Specialist Quality Assurance, City and Hackney Provider Unit

Kevin Hope, BSc(Hons), RGN, RMN, Cert Ed, RNT
Nurse Tutor, Stockport, Tameside and Glossop College of Nursing

Penny Irwin, BA, RGN, SCM, MSc
Senior Nurse Quality Assurance, City and Hackney Provider Unit

Joan Kemp, BA(Hons), MSc, M Phil, RGN, RCNT, RNT
Lecturer in Nursing Studies, University of Hull

Richard McMahon, MA, Dip N, RGN
Senior Nurse Elderly Care, Horton General Hospital, and Lecturer Practitioner, Oxford Polytechnic

Lawrence Smith, BA(Hons), PhD
Research Scientist, MRC/ESRC Social and Applied Psychology Unit, University of Sheffield

Peter Totterdell, BSc, MSc
Research Officer, MRC/ESRC Social and Applied Psychology Unit, University of Sheffield

Fiona Wilkinson, RGN, Dip N(Wales), RNT
Independent Health Care Management Consultant

Chapter 1
Introduction:
What's So Special
About Nursing at Night?
Richard McMahon

Introduction

This book has been written for nurses: not only permanent night nurses or nurses who work internal rotation, but all nurses who care for patients, who manage a service which includes caring at night or who are involved in nurse education. This may seem an ambitious claim; however, the philosophy behind this book is based on some fundamental assumptions. For example, it is now well recognised that nurses should care holistically for their patients, taking into account individual social, psychological and normal physical characteristics as well as illness and treatment-related factors. The logical extension of this is the realisation that a person's day- and night-time functioning are interdependent, and that this can become crucial for the well-being of hospital patients.

Yet night nursing has for a long time been considered a caretaking service requiring no particular expertise, and which has in many hospitals provided a destination for errant nurses where they could supposedly do the minimum of damage. This book demonstrates that there are many aspects of caring at night which are unique and which require specialist knowledge and attention; this fact needs to be appreciated by all members of the nursing team, including those practising in the day, in management, and in education.

Whilst this book is aimed at all nurses, it is recognised and expected that it will be read predominantly by those who work either all or some of their shifts during the hours of darkness. Therefore much of the material presented is aimed at highlighting the issues related to these nurses, and bearing in mind that this group is frequently disadvantaged (both socially and at work) when it comes to opportunities for self-development.

Following this preliminary chapter which examines some of the broad issues relating to night nurses, this book has been roughly divided in two. The first half deals mainly with clinical issues such as pain and sleep, the second with broader aspects of care such as education and quality assurance. The book concludes with a chapter looking forward to how night nursing, and the lot of night nurses, may be developed in the future.

This chapter aims to describe some of the issues which surround night nursing practice. It is largely based on anecdotal evidence accumulated from the attenders from all over the country on night nurses' study days which have been running for the last three years. The purpose of this chapter is not to judge any of the issues raised, or to suggest solutions. Instead, the issues are presented to give an overview of what we know about current night nursing so that the rest of the book can be placed in context. Ideas for some options for a way forward for night nursing may be found in the final chapter.

This particular chapter has a number of themes. Firstly, to describe ways in which patients are different at night compared with during the day. After all, they are the same individuals, so it is not necessarily self-evident that they have different needs at night. Secondly, the night shift presents many problems physically, mentally and socially for those that work it, yet many night nurses feel extremely positive about their experiences of night work (Watson 1982, Janowski 1988). Next, some of the findings from the Department of Health and Social Security's (DHSS) multi-centre survey of night nursing services are discussed. This is followed by a description of some of the current political issues that particularly relate to night nurses. Finally, the chapter finishes by presenting some of the challenges to nursing in providing a caring service at night.

What's Different at Night for the Patients?

If the needs of patients at night were identical to those in the day, there really would be little need for this book. However, night-time produces new problems and different emphases for pre-existing ones. Unfortunately, there is a dearth of research to confirm or question the significance of many of the issues raised here.

Sleep

Clearly one of the principal goals for the majority of patients with the onset of darkness is to get what they judge to be a satisfactory night's sleep. Those caring at night need to be experts *par excellence* in promoting and maintaining sleep, as there is considerable evidence that patients in hospital suffer sleep disturbance (Wilson-Barnett 1978, Closs 1988). Unfortunately, many nurses are unaware of the physiology of sleep and types of sleeplessness. The nursing response to the sleepless patient has for too long been to resort to drugs, as this provides an easy solution for the nurse and a recognisable and short-term solution for the patient.

However, an increasing number of nurses now understand the problems associated with the benzodiazepines and other artificial sleep inducing substances. There is a greater recognition that nurses and the surrounding environment are a major source of disturbance for patients (Ogilvie 1980) and that there are a large number of non-pharmacological interventions which night nurses may adopt (McMahon 1990a).

Mental Well-being

Many people experience the phenomenon of being reasonably cheerful whilst active during the day, only to experience a disproportionate level of anxiety and fear at night in bed. How much this may be exaggerated for a patient the night before an operation, or if he fears or knows that he has a terminal disease, or that he will never be able to live in his own home again, is something that can only be guessed at by many nurses. Even when there is no major focus, patients may experience simple boredom or loneliness. Nurses caring at night not only need the skills to assess the mental states of their patients, but also require the skills to intervene in an effective way; be it by offering the patient the radio headset, or enough time over a number of nights to build up the confidence and courage to express his fears. Stress and anxiety also have a major bearing on the individual's ability to get to sleep (Johns et al 1974).

Another problem confronted by night nurses is increased disturbed behaviour by confused patients. Some patients only exhibit confusional states at night, whilst for some that are permanently disorientated, the twilight hours seem to prompt an increase in wandering and agitation, probably at least partially due to the sensory deprivation created by dimming the lights (Cameron, cited in Chadwick 1984).

Changes in Functional Ability

There are many reasons why patients may be less able to care for themselves at night compared with their abilities in the day. Factors such as dim lighting making the patient unsure of his movements, tiredness, the 'hangover' effects of sleeping tablets, and unfamiliar or unhelpful furniture may all contribute to an increased level of dependence. In certain client groups, such as the elderly, the overcoming of such hurdles can make the difference between discharge to the patient's own home or discharge to an institution, as few community services extend into the night. Night nurses need to be as skilled as day-time nurses in such activities as teaching patients to transfer from a bed to a chair.

What Makes Night Nursing Special for the Nurses?

Nurses who work regular nights report many factors that make the clinical work they do different from daytime activities. Some of these reflect the satisfaction derived from night work, whilst others present difficulties.

More Time for Patients as People

It has been well documented that on most wards at night the most frenetic activity occurs in the first and last two hours of the shift (NHS Management Consultancy Services 1987). The middle of the night tends to have less activity, a time which coincides with the period when patients experiencing sleeplessness due to anxiety for whatever reason can benefit from the company of a nurse. Macleod-Clark (1983) has shown that much nursing communication revolves around some form of physical intervention, it would be interesting to investigate if the same is true at night.

As part of providing psychological support, nurses comment that they are able to allay fears through teaching the patients on an individual basis about their health, illnesses, investigations and treatments.

The Need to be Vigilant and Adaptable

Night nurses report that they find it extremely challenging that, at a time when they are often at a low ebb physically, they are expected to assess and respond to unpredictable situations, with fewer resources on the ward and less back-up from non-nursing services. For example, nursing research (Thompson et al 1985) has indicated that the most common time for patients to suffer chest pain and myocardial infarction is during the night.

Teamwork and Comradeship

In hospitals where a permanent night staff is the norm, it is not uncommon for nurses to feel part of two teams;

  (i) the ward team where the other team members are only seen at handover, but where the patients are a common link, and
  (ii) the team of night nurses where the common link is each other.

Night nurses often feel that there is a strong team spirit on night duty, and that this is heightened when there is a crisis as the nurses only have each other to help them. Also, the common experience of the difficulties of shift work can lead to a team spirit extending beyond nursing to other disciplines and occupations.

Management and Problem-solving Experience

Up until the mid 1980s, it was not uncommon for student nurses to get their first taste of 'in charge' experience on night duty. That practice has all but been abandoned, yet qualified night nurses feel that they have a large managerial component in their work. Night nurses feel that they have to problem-solve using creativity and ingenuity to overcome challenges without the back-up available in the day. However, in many areas such as the large teaching hospitals, night sisters' posts are used as training posts for day sisters' posts; the managerial responsibilities of night staff do not seem to be recognised or valued on their own merits.

Social Necessity and Advantages

Many nurses who work permanent night duty do so for the simple reason that they have to work for financial reasons, and night duty fits in with their family commitments. As the night duty is currently longer than traditional day shifts, then working time can be concentrated into the fewest possible number of occurrences. The relatively long periods of time off duty between periods of shifts is attractive to occasional and permanent night nurses alike. Another advantage cited by many night nurses is travel against the main flow of traffic and often easier parking at the hospital.

What Happens at Night?

One of the difficulties about describing care at night is that it is only recently that there has been any significant level of research activity in the field. The most extensive work describing current activity in hospitals at night was published by the DHSS in 1987. This descriptive work attempted to provide a profile of many aspects of night nursing in district general hospitals (DGHs) based on field research in 4 wards in each of 10 hospitals and questionnaire responses from these and 30 other DGHs.

The DHSS study (NHS Management Consultancy Services 1987) made a number of interesting observations (Table 1.1) many of which give a useful insight into the night nursing service.

Table 1.1 A summary of selected observations from DHSS study of night nursing services (NHS Management Consultancy Services 1987)

---

   i. In general, there was no established way of setting and monitoring standards at night. There nursing service was required to provide a good standard of care, without any method of knowing what a good standard was or whether it was being achieved.
   ii. 82% of the general wards surveyed had 3 or more nurses on duty each night.
   iii. Trained nurses were in charge of wards 99.3% of the time, with two or more trained nurses being present 52.8% of the time.
   iv. At night care tended to become task-orientated, despite other methods of work allocation on the ward in the day.
   v. Trained nurses spent most of their time with patients, or performing activities related to patient care.
   vi. 6am drug rounds persisted, despite an over-riding professional opinion that this was inappropriate.
   vii. 82.4% of night sisters felt that their security needs were not fully met.
   viii. 80% of nurses in the postal sample felt that their professional needs were being met because they felt that night duty provided them with greater managerial experience and added responsibility.
   ix. However, most night nurses seemed to be disadvantaged in management and clinical training.
   x. Night nurses provide a largely reactive, demand led service.

Quality Assurance

The DHSS report commented on the lack of quality assurance initiatives at night. The recent trend to examine the quality of care received by patients (Pearson 1987) using established tools seems to have rarely permeated through to care at night. Nurses have in the past discussed the standards of care at night without agreeing any common criteria to judge those standards. For example, a ward on which all the patients have had a wash and been put in their chairs before the morning shift arrive may be interpreted as giving a high standard of care by one nurse, and a poor standard by another. How can one say that standards are improving or dropping as a result of a change, if what constitutes good care has not been established?

Rather than rushing to develop quality assurance tools and programmes that incorporate night care more effectively, there is an initiative to set standard of care based on the Dynamic Standard Setting System developed by the Royal College of Nursing (Kitson 1989). This approach, an example of which appears in Chapter 9, has some distinct advantages. Firstly, it is a method which is about nurses on the wards looking at quality, rather than managers examining areas in a critical and often pejorative way. Secondly, the level of care set as a desirable standard is agreed by a group of peers through discussion and argument. Thirdly, it is specifically a problem-solving tool; by setting standards in areas of practice perceived to be problematic, the nurses have to come up with workable solutions to those problems. Finally, the system demands that achievable and measurable criteria are set so that the quality can be monitored.

Number of Nurses on Duty at Night

The days when one nurse was left on duty at night in a medical or surgical ward have long gone. Since the middle of the century the increase in the level of medical activity (in terms of complexity, use of technology and throughput) has been almost exponential, and the consequent demands on nursing have paralleled that rise. The research by the DHSS found that most general wards had three or more nurses on duty at night. The relationship between the level of activity on a ward and the number and skill-mix of nurses required to provide a quality service is coming under close scrutiny under current government initiatives.

Proportion of Trained Nurses

Over the last 10 years a greater appreciation has developed of the responsibilities and accountability of the trained nurse, along with a re-evaluation of the role of nurse learners. The DHSS found trained nurses to be on duty on almost all the wards. Just over half the wards had two or more trained nurses at night.

Perpetuation of Task Allocation

The NHS Management Consultancy Service reported that although patient allocation and other ward management systems have become widespread, they found that night care tended to be organised around task allocation. Where there is only one trained nurse on duty, it is easy to see how there must be a division of labour to the extent that there are certain tasks which only a trained nurse can perform, such as the administration of medicines. However, whatever the mix of qualified and unqualified nurses, the principles of patient allocation can be achieved to an acceptable degree. The reasons why task allocation has been retained at night may only be guessed at, but it would seem self-evident that one factor is that night staff do not benefit from the same level of support and development as their day-time colleagues.

Caring for Patients

The report clearly showed that caring for patients was a major role for trained nurses. Unlike their day-time colleagues who got involved in ward rounds and coordinating activity on the ward, qualified nurses at night mainly performed the role they had been trained for, that is, nursing patients.

Drug Rounds

The performing of a drug round at 6am was still a widespread practice, about which the report stated that:

'. . . the overwhelming professional opinion of senior nurse managers and night nurses was that in most cases the current practice of rousing patients at 06.00 hours to take medication on an empty stomach was unnecessary, inappropriate, and contrary to the philosophy of personalised patient care.' (NHS Management Consultancy Services 1989)

This apparent contradiction reflects the stagnation in many areas to allow a poor practice to continue despite opposition at all levels. The reasons for this are hard to identify; however, poor communication is one likely contributory factor.

Security Needs

The media regularly reports attacks on hospital staff and patients. Night sisters are often required to move around the hospital at night, an activity which may involve going outside which can often be a frightening experience. However, if great expense has been spent on security, as in complex buildings such as hospitals, this involves the utilisation of both technology and manpower. To what extent the provision of security is viewed as a necessity as opposed to a luxury may well depend on an atrocity actually occurring within the hospital.

Professional Needs

Four-fifths of the postal sample felt that their professional needs were being met through night work. The main sources of this satisfaction seemed to be the greater managerial role and degree of responsibility they perceived to be vested in them. It is encouraging that night nurses felt that they were getting good managerial experience, as their managerial responsibilities are different from their day-time colleagues'. For example, night nurses, including sisters, are not often involved by day colleagues in budgeting, attending meetings, negotiating or the recruiting and dismissing of staff although they are often willing to do so. Instead the type of management experience night nurses get is in such areas as working without direct supervision, decision making, 'man' management and monitoring standards.

Training

Whilst night nurses got satisfaction out of the managerial aspects of their job, the project reported that night nurses seemed to be disadvantaged when it came to management training. Similarly, in clinical subjects night nurses found it hard to gain access to courses. This can be attributed to a number of factors. Firstly, many night nurses have difficulty attending activities in the day, this being the reason why they chose night work. Secondly, managers are often reluctant to send night nurses as they feel that they are not a priority group and because finding a replacement nurse can be difficult at night. Thirdly, many night nurses have not had the necessary development which helps individuals to recognise their own learning needs, and hence take responsibility for their own further development.

A Reactive and Demand Led Service

This is a perceptive and telling comment on the service. Whilst to some extent all general nursing is reactive and demand led, in the case of night nursing this has been particularly true. Yet, much of the thrust of current nursing innovation is about assessing and predicting patients' needs and planning care. All too often it seems that the period of night duty revolves around one of two ends of a continuum. At one end is the highly organised and task-related approach, in which nurses systematically go from bed to bed, turning, toileting or offering some other aspect of care to each patient. At the other end is the approach which is highly reactive, with the nurses moving between the patients they perceive to be in the greatest need and those who are able to attract the most attention.

The solution to the comment of being reactive and demand led lies in two initiatives. The first is to have organised management that predicts and plans for rises and falls in dependency, and which responds with appropriate staffing levels. The second is for the nurses to spend more time planning and negotiating with their patients, and keeping them informed about care. By anticipating needs for analgesia, support or perhaps elimination, the nurse is able to pre-empt demands on her at a later stage. However, to reach the stage where the nurse can accurately anticipate needs, she needs to have knowledge of the field she is working in, knowledge of her individual patients, and the skills to prioritise and make decisions about the management of care.

Clearly the DHSS study provided a wealth of information as a result of which the Department of Health is now sponsoring three more research projects investigating further issues relating to nursing at night.

Two of the studies are being carried out at the Nuffield Institute for Health Services Studies at the University of Leeds. The first study is examining patients' experiences of care at night, something that the original study did not address. The project will also examine nurses' opinions of the organisation of care at night and the obstructions to change. The second study is considering the role of night sisters/charge nurses and night nursing service managers. As will become clear in the next section of this chapter, the issue of how night nursing is managed is becoming the subject of considerable debate.

The third study commissioned by the Department of Health, which is being undertaken by Simon Folkard and his team (see Chapter 8), is looking in detail at the effects of shiftwork on night nurses, and how variables such as number of nights worked or the length of shift influences the problems experienced by night nurses.

Together, these three studies will help to clarify further the picture we have of night nursing.

Political Issues in Night Nursing

As with any identifiable group within an organisation, there are various issues relating to power which affect that group. At the present time, night nursing services seem to be being directly affected by the changes that continue to pass through the Health Service.

The Role of the Night Sister

In general, the role of the night sister has been of a peripatetic adviser, manager and helper. However, changes in the ways hospitals and nursing are managed are eroding the night sister's role.

The move away from a centrally held budget which paid for a 'pool' of night nurses to a developed system in which the staff and money are the responsibility of the ward sister has resulted in a situation whereby the nurse in charge of a ward at night nearly always knows the ward and the speciality extremely well. This, in association with cessation of the use of learners in charge of wards at night, has clarified the issue of accountability and has reduced the need for a visiting adviser and supervisor. In many districts, this has led to nearly all the nurses previously funded under the 'night' budget becoming ward based. This has had at least two effects. Firstly, it has led to the move away from the identification by individuals with the 'hospital night staff' to identification with the 'ward night staff'. Unfortunately, it seems that only rarely has this move led to an identification with the 'ward staff' without the creation of a sub-group. Secondly, it has meant a move to a more clinical role with far less managerial responsibility. The consequence of this second effect has been that as night sisters leave, they are being replaced with staff who have neither the title nor the grade of their predecessors.

Accountability for Care at Night

Major changes have occurred in the way nursing care is managed. With the advent of team, and in particular primary nursing, there has been a delegation of accountability away from the ward sister to individual staff nurses for the care of individual patients (Pearson 1988). In the past, the day staff in many places were perceived to be accountable for care during the day, and night staff for care at night, and that the two rarely tried to influence each other, the only exception being that of the ward sister who reigned supreme over both. With many of the new approaches to care, day-time primary nurses and team leaders have a responsibility to plan their patients' care for when they are not on duty, including at night. This has been viewed by some night nurses as a tiresome meddling in their affairs and interpreted by others as a loss of status and power, particularly if the day-time care planner is 'junior' either in years or grade. However, many night nurses have recognised that the motivation for this change is to enable the patient to benefit from consistent care which can be evaluated, and that accountability for decision making must rest with an identifiable individual. Unfortunately, not only is the purpose and functioning of systems such as primary nursing misunderstood by some night nurses (e.g. Remington 1989), but also by day nurses working within the system. This may result in the contribution that the night nurse has to make in the assessing and planning of care being devalued or even ignored. The correct implementation of primary nursing is to develop collegial relations between members of staff, thus promoting respect, trust and understanding based on the valuing of each other's previous experience, training and values (McMahon 1990b).

The Challenge to Nursing

Much of this chapter has focused on the clinical and political issues surrounding caring at night. If nursing is to provide a high quality service to patients, a number of fundamental problems must be addressed.

Lack of Research

Much of the evidence for statements made in this chapter arises from the accounts given by night nurses themselves. There is a desperate need for systematic enquiry into the ways in which patients' needs alter at night, and what the best nursing responses to these changes might be. If nursing does not identify specialist needs at night the 'caretaking' image will persist, with the possibility of the need for more than one trained nurse being required on night duty being questioned by general managers or under Resource Management, Clinical Management Teams or Directorates.

Maximising Performance

It is well documented that shift workers perform less well at night compared with their day-time abilities (Folkard and Monk 1985). However, nurses need to be vigilant, resourceful and accurate both at night and during the day. If carers at night are to provide a safe and effective night nursing service, then the service must respond to knowledge about the effects of shiftwork. For example, in many hospitals it is common practice for fluid balance charts to be added up at midnight or, worse, at 7am. Such practices are inviting mistakes. Similarly, research into identifying those who are particularly suited and unsuited to night duty has been in progress for some time (Folkard et al 1979), and recent work (Alward and Monk 1990) has indicated that a successful change to night work may relate more to social rather than biological adjustment.

Nurses at Night Becoming Proactive, Therapeutic Nurses

There are several factors that need resolution if nursing is to respond to this challenge. Firstly, nurses have to overcome the perception that patient care at night is trivial. More nurses need to demonstrate through their actions a genuine belief in the concept of holism, and hence that patients' physical and mental well-being are related, and that day and night-time abilities and degree of wellness are inextricably linked. Secondly, nursing needs to investigate which of its established interventions actually benefit the patient at night, and also develop innovative new ones. This should involve many aspects of nursing care including the effective use of interpersonal skills, physical interventions and patient teaching. For example, it would seem that an increase in periods of wakefulness at night along with more daytime napping is a characteristic of normal ageing (Hayter 1983). An elderly patient complaining of sleeplessness may, in fact, be having a 'normal' experience requiring an educative response from the nurse, rather than one aimed at producing a sleep pattern characteristic of younger adults.

Bridging the Day-Night Divide

It is undoubtedly true that in many wards and departments that provide care overnight there is a degree of tension between those seen to be 'day' and 'night' nurses. This situation is not new; however, it is divisive and destructive. The time has come in modern nursing to confront this problem head on, and as a consequence, start working more effectively in collaborative relationships.

Redressing the Imbalance in Training and Other Facilities Available to Nurses Working Different Shifts

Many current issues in nursing have a direct bearing on this challenge. The forthcoming requirement for nurses to demonstrate that they are at least maintaining their level of knowledge and skill if they are to stay on the register, media reports of frequent physical attacks on hospital staff and patients, potential recruitment problems as a result of the 'demographic time-bomb' and many other factors make the need for change increasingly urgent.

Retaining Expertise and a Career Structure for Night Nurses

The current trend towards moving resources away from night nursing has already been examined. Management units need to make decisions as to how to proceed with care at night. Where a permanent night team is retained, a drain of resources will lead to a drain of skill and experience at a time when the needs of patients at night are becoming more widely recognised. Equally, a move to internal rotation ignores the social reasons that make many nurses choose night work, again leading to a loss of valuable personnel. Creative solutions are required if the multiple influences on staff retention are to be effectively managed.

Conclusion

Providing care at night makes unique demands on nurses both clinically and personally. However, for many historical as well as practical and financial reasons the people who nurse at night are disadvantaged in educational opportunities, facilities and status. Current innovations in the management of care are perceived by many night nurses as further undermining their position, and the day staff–night staff divide seems to be a tenacious problem despite the espousing of the concepts of holism and patient-centred care.

However, regardless of whether wards are staffed with permanent night staff or operate a system of internal rotation, there is a body of both clinical and professional knowledge which is of relevance to anyone caring for in-patients at night. This book is about starting to bring that knowledge together in one place for the benefit of patients. If, as a side effect, this assists in the raising of the value accorded to care at night and those who give it then this is to the good. At the end of the day, it should be our aim to have a very high awareness of patients' problems at night, how they relate to day-time functioning and events, and how they might be solved, whilst at the same time completely removing any distinction between those who provide the care in the day and at night.

References

Alward R R and Monk T H (1990) A comparison of rotating-shift and permanent night nurses. *International Journal of Nursing Studies*, **27**, 3, 297–302.

Armstrong M (1987) No proper time of day. *Occupational Health*, **39**, 2, 54–56.

Chadwick P (1984) Social stimulation and the elderly. *Nursing Times*, **80**, 10, 41–42.

Closs S J (1988) *A Nursing Study of Sleep on Surgical Wards*. University of Edinburgh Department of Nursing Studies.

Folkard S and Monk T H (eds) (1985) *Hours of Work: Temporal Factors in Work Scheduling*. Chichester: John Wiley.

Folkard S, Monk T H and Lobban M C (1979) Towards a predictive test of adjustment to shiftwork. *Ergonomics*, **22**, 1, 79–91.

Hayter J (1983) Sleep behaviours of older persons. *Nursing Research*, **32**, 242–246.

Janowski M J (1988) More from the night owls. *American Journal of Nursing*, **88**, 10, 1340–1341.

Johns M W, Bruce D W and Masterton J P (1974) Psychological correlates of sleep habits reported by healthy young adults. *British Journal of Medical Psychology*, **47**, 181–187.

Kitson A (1989) *A Framework for Quality*. London: RCN.

Macleod-Clark J (1983) Nurse-patient communication – an analysis of conversations from surgical wards. In, Wilson-Barnett, J (ed) *Nursing Research: Ten Studies in Patient Care*. Chichester: John Wiley.

McMahon R (1990a) Sleep therapies. *Surgical Nurse*, **3**, 5, 17–20.

McMahon R (1990b) Collegiality is the key. *Nursing Times*, **86**, 42, 66–67.

NHS Management Consultancy Services (1987) *Study of Night Nursing Services*. London: DHSS.

Ogilvie A J (1980) Sources and levels of noise on the ward at night. *Nursing Times*, **76**, 31, 1363–66.

Pearson A (ed) (1987) *Nursing Quality Measurement*, Chichester: John Wiley.

Pearson A (ed) (1988) *Primary Nursing: The Work of the Burford and Oxford Nursing Development Unit*. London: Croom Helm.

Remington J (1989) Primary nursing: night rites. *Nursing Times*, **85**, 1, 30–31.

Thompson D R, Blandford R L, Sutton T W and Marchant P R (1985) Time of onset of chest pain in acute myocardial infarction. *International Journal of Cardiology*, **7**, 139–146.

Watson C (1982) Sleepless night, peaceful night. *Nursing Mirror*, **155**, 11, 22.

Wilson-Barnett J (1978) In hospital: patient's feelings and opinions. *Nursing Times (Occasional Paper)*, **74**, 11, 29–34.

Chapter 2
Assessing the Individual at Night
Penny Irwin

Introduction

The assessment of the patient at night cannot be divorced from the holistic assessment which should have occurred on admission and shortly afterwards. Whilst the initial assessment of the patient may have been carried out in the day-time, the night staff should also add their contribution as a result of their experience and observation of the patient during the night. The role of the nurse at night is very involved with patients' sleep and the events which may disturb it. Sleep, as later chapters will show, is an important part of all patients' comfort, well-being and recovery, but has not been given the nursing priority it deserves. This chapter will look at ways in which nurses can effectively assess and evaluate patients' sleep, and problems during the night.

No particular model of nursing will be suggested in the course of this discussion, rather it is hoped that the principles of assessment in relation to sleep and disturbed sleep patterns can be incorporated into whatever model is being used.

Sleep in Hospital

The need that the sick have for sleep was well recognised by Florence Nightingale:

> 'Never to allow a patient to be waked, intentionally or accidentally, is a *"sine qua non"* of all good nursing.' (Nightingale 1859, p 33)

Unfortunately there is much research to show that patients are sleep-deprived in hospital. Environmental factors, such as noise, lighting, ambient temperature and ward routine, are significant causes (Murphy et al 1977, Dodds 1980, Carter 1984, Closs 1988). Sleep research has also shown that different illnesses disrupt sleep in characteristic ways. There are therefore many reasons why patients may not sleep in hospital. This might well be recognised and accepted as the norm, but as nurses we should be aware that sleep deprivation can be detrimental to patients' comfort and well-being in the day-time. Irritability and lethargy are perhaps some of the better known symptoms, but recent research indicates that there are others. Importantly, unexplained generalised musculo-skeletal pains have been shown to occur in any condition whatever the cause of the sleep deprivation (Moldofsky 1986, Moldofsky et al 1987). Florence Nightingale was therefore right when she said:

'Pain, like irritability of brain, perpetuates and intensifies itself. If you have gained a respite of either in sleep you have gained more than the mere respite. Both the probability of recurrence and of the same intensity will be diminished; whereas both will be terribly increased by want of sleep.' (Nightingale 1859, p 34)

Issues in Nursing Assessment and Management of Patients' Sleep

Nursing research indicates that nurses inadequately assess patients' sleep needs or properly evaluate their sleep difficulties (Closs 1988, Carter 1984, Dodds 1980). Night staff have traditionally been regarded as 'care-takers' and seen themselves as lower status to the day staff (Kemp 1984). This has affected their contribution to the team assessment and evaluation of patient care, for if there is no mechanism for their information to be included in the patient's assessment, or the likelihood is that it will be disregarded by the day staff anyway, then it is not surprising if they are tempted not to communicate it. If there is internal rotation to nights in operation, communication may improve, but even so patient problems that have manifest themselves at night and which need action in the day can still remain unresolved.

Part of the problem has been the lack of knowledge staff have about sleep. It has been well recognised that the nursing literature has until recently failed to bring the knowledge about sleep into the nursing arena (Kemp 1984). Unfortunately, the knowledge coming from the sleep researchers in such abundance is in journals related to the specific disciplines in which the research was conducted, such as medicine, psychology, physiology and biochemistry. It takes a while for this to be translated into the nursing literature. Nurses can therefore be working in ignorance of what is a scientifically well-accepted fact for several years. Hopefully this will be remedied in part by this book and nurses will see that we have much to catch up in the area of sleep assessment and evaluation.

The Principles of Assessment

Assessment, as the first stage in the nursing process, is the systematic collection of information regarding the patient's health and factors which affect it. From this information the nurse, using her knowledge base, can identify problems which require nursing intervention (i.e. make nursing diagnoses). The nurse at night, therefore, requires a knowledge of all aspects of care, and in particular, sleep and its relationship to physical, psychological and disease states in order to effectively assess the patient and plan appropriate interventions.

The process of assessment involves one or more interviews with the patient (and/or his family), physical examination, observation, review of previous records and, very often, discussion with other members of the multi-disciplinary team (Carpenito 1989, Hunt and Marks-Maran 1986). Factors taken into account in any nursing assessment no matter what its framework include maturational, environmental, personal, patho-physiological and treatment-related factors. Knowledge of all these is important in understanding the individual.

Night-time behaviour and symptoms can be very different to the day, so the night nursing assessment can highlight different aspects of the patient's illness and his responses to it. This adds an important dimension to the total assessment, which should enhance the total plan of care. Some symptoms are worse at night than they are in the day. Confusion in the elderly is often worse at night; whilst the depressed patient may reach his lowest ebb in the early dawn hours. Anxiety about a pending operation may manifest itself in sleeplessness. Physical weaknesses might also be more evident in the middle of the night when sleepiness can lead to lack of co-ordination. Nearing the time for discharge home, the night assessment will have an important part to play in the total decisions about patient discharge. It is very often crucial to the successful discharge home of some patients that they are able to look after themselves, at night as well as during the day. How the patient manages to walk to the toilet, or transfer from bed to commode at 3 o'clock in the morning, may be very different to how he copes at the same time in the afternoon.

No assessment should be done without including the patient's sleep pattern, particularly at night. Little exists in nursing to enable this to be done systematically. However, methods used by sleep research workers to assess and evaluate sleep have been well proven and could be incorporated into the nursing assessment and evaluation of patients' sleep with very little trouble because they are so simple. If nurses routinely used such methods they would be able to communicate patients' sleep difficulties to each other in a consistent, meaningful way, which could result in the more effective management of the problems identified. These methods are described below.

Initial Assessment Details Regarding Patients' Night-Time Habits and Sleep Patterns

Human sleep patterns have been shown to vary with age, sex, genetics and upbringing, environment and illness. Variations in the length of time people need to sleep varies from five to nine hours. This is not necessarily dependent on the amount of stress and activity undertaken (Horne 1988), but may be just what that individual needs. Illness has effects related to aetiology and symptoms which may disturb sleep or create a greater need. It is therefore important to be mindful of all these factors when assessing the patient and his sleep pattern.

Sleep Assessment – The Observable Features of Sleep

The observable features of sleep have been used for some time by sleep researchers in conjunction with sleep Electro-encephalogram (EEG) studies (Bixler and Vela Bueno 1989). In these studies it has been demonstrated that people's subjective reports of their sleep quality the morning after they have slept have correlated well with their sleep EEG (Carskadon et al 1976, Frankel et al 1976, Johns 1977, Johns and Doré 1978). The most common discrepancy in normal subjects between reported and objective data seems to be that morning estimates of awakenings during the night are underestimated when compared to their EEG recordings (Sewitch 1984). These same features of sleep also serve as useful measurements in studies which do not use EEG, but other techniques, such as questionnaires. They could also be adopted for use in the routine nursing assessment and evaluation of patients' sleep. They are described in Table 2.1.

Table 2.1 Sleep assessment tool: the observable features of sleep (Bixler and Vela Bueno 1987, Closs 1988, Parkes 1985)

1. *Settling down time*	– Going to bed time.
2. *Sleep onset time*	– Time when the individual goes to sleep.
3. *Sleep onset latency (SOL)*	– The time between the settling down time and the sleep onset time.
4. *Number of night awakenings*	– and their duration. (In nursing it would be important to know the reasons for waking, and what helps the patient go off to sleep again.)
5. *Morning waking time*	– Time when the individual wakes in the morning.
6. *Total sleep time (TST)*	– The total time spent asleep from sleep onset to finally waking up in the morning. (Wakings in the night in EEG studies can be timed and subtracted from the sleep time, so that only time spent sleeping is included. In nursing this is difficult and could only be approximated.)
7. *Time in bed (TIB)*	– Time in bed from settling at night to getting up in the morning.
8. *Sleep efficiency*	– An index of Total Sleep Time as a proportion of Time in Bed (assuming the person is trying to sleep). This is often expressed as a percentage.
	i.e. $\dfrac{\text{Total sleep time}}{\text{Time in bed}} \times 100$
9. *Day-time naps*	– Sleep during the day (which should be included in the total sleep time for the 24 hours).

Patient Assessment

The patient's biographical details will enable the nurse to form a picture of him as an individual, and also give important information related to their sleep pattern.

Age

Sleep varies with age. As people grow older so their sleep time becomes shorter and the sleep cycle (to be described in later chapters) is affected. The elderly are known to have more night wakings (often to go to the toilet) and to wake early in the morning (Borbély 1986, Morgan 1987). Because of the different rate at which people respond to the ageing process, it is not possible to be exact about the age at which changes in sleep pattern occur. Hayter (1983) in a study of the elderly from 65 years of age upwards noted that the main changes in going to bed times, time in bed, time awake during the night and day-time naps occurred after the age of 75 years. The total sleep time for subjects 75 years and over gradually increased owing to the number of day-time naps they took, and this difference was even more marked in the age group over 85 years old.

Therefore, assessment of the elderly patient, in particular, should take into account the day-time naps they are used to taking. It may well be that these form an important part of their total sleep time, that they lie awake in bed for some time in the night as a result and often want to get up very early in the morning.

Gender

Women are more likely to consult their doctor about insomnia (Borbély 1986) and studies show they consume far more sleeping tablets than men (Murray et al 1981). However, repeated studies show that men have more disturbed sleep than women at all ages (Closs 1988, Horne 1988, Webb 1982), so men may underestimate the sleep disturbance they have.

Living Alone

Dodds (1980) found that patients who lived alone reported that they slept better in hospital. She attributed this to the alleviation of worry about their symptoms and what might happen if they were on their own in the event of an acute exacerbation. Closs (1988) also found that patients who lived alone at home compared their sleep in hospital more favourably than those who lived with others. This is not to say that all patients who live alone will sleep better in hospital, but it does say that many of them find great comfort in the presence of nurses to provide help and comfort in the event of exacerbated and frightening symptoms.

Customary Sleep Pattern

The patient's normal sleep pattern at home will have an important bearing on his sleep in hospital. Those who usually sleep badly at home may be expected to do so in hospital, whereas those who sleep well at home but not in hospital will need assessing as to what the reasons might be. The use of the sleep assessment tool described above will elicit important information to enable the nurse to plan care to facilitate the patient's sleep in hospital.

What Time Does the Patient Normally Go to Bed at Night?

The time people normally go to bed at night varies with the individual. Hone and Ostberg (1976) proved that some people are 'morning types', who go to bed early and wake up early in the morning full of energy. By contrast 'evening types' like to stay up late, are the 'life and soul of the party', and wake up late in the morning. The 'evening type' will generally feel sleep deprived if he wakes up early. It is not known if these differences between people are inherited or result from their life-style. Whatever the cause, it is understandable that patients coming into hospital will find it difficult to adapt to a set time for going to bed if they are used to something very different, whether it be earlier or later. Ideally the ward routine should facilitate patients' settling down for the night in their own time.

Pre-Sleep Routines

The routines people follow before settling down to sleep help them relax. Pre-sleep routines have been proven by some researchers to be correlated with a better night's sleep, particularly in the elderly (Johnson 1986). Some patients may settle following a routine alcoholic drink, or a cigarette. Others may like to read for a while, whilst others prefer a milky drink.

A research study in the early 1970s showed that milky drinks before going to bed or after night wakings helped people go to sleep more easily (Brezinova and Oswald 1972). This study was criticised for many reasons but there may be a physiological basis for milky drinks having this effect. Milk contains L-tryptophan (a precursor of serotonin which is thought to be one of the substances involved in the onset of sleep), which when given intravenously has been shown to reduce sleep onset latency and the number of night awakenings, and give a better rated quality of sleep (Korner 1986). The evidence for oral L-tryptophan is not so conclusive. Nonetheless, patients may well find a milky drink before they settle for the night very comforting, particularly if they are accustomed to it.

Does the Patient Have Any Difficulties with Going to Sleep?

Any difficulties going to sleep, which cause a prolonged sleep onset latency, may often be related to symptoms of the patient's illness, but anxiety, environmental factors and unexplained insomnia may also be reasons. Anxiety is associated with a prolonged sleep onset latency and many night awakenings. Wilson-Barnett and Carrigy (1978) highlighted the association between a major test and medical patients' anxiety levels. They found anxiety scores on the day of major tests were significantly higher than for other days in hospital. Borbély (1986) indicates from studies in Switzerland that the most frequently named cause of being unable to sleep given was people being unable to get thoughts out of their head. Beszterczey (1977) demonstrated in a study of cancer patients that insomnia in these patients was positively correlated with anxiety and depression, rather than with pain.

How Often Does the Patient Wake in the Night?

If patients have been ill for some time before they come into hospital their sleep may be disrupted with constant night awakenings because of their symptoms. Someone who normally sleeps well may not have done so for several weeks or months because of their symptoms. Very often they have developed important coping strategies at home (such as sleeping with several pillows for indigestion or breathlessness), which if known about, can be incorporated into their nursing care in hospital. The nurse, therefore, should spend some time discussing with the patient why he wakes at night, and if anything in particular helps him to sleep better.

Carter (1984) found that the main reasons for medical patients' sleep disturbance were physical, such as dyspnoea and pain. Many of the patients in this study, and that by Irwin (1989), found their sleep improved on coming into hospital because their symptoms were better controlled, showing that patients put up with considerable discomfort at home.

Any symptoms which cause discomfort will cause the patient to wake in the night or for their sleep to be disturbed. These include:

Pain	Obstructive sleep apnoea/snoring
Cramps	Nocturia
Itching	Enuresis/discomfort from incontinence
Indigestion	Bowel discomfort
Dyspnoea	Nightmares
Coughing	Anxiety/fear/worry
Palpitations	Depression

The interventions for patient problems at night will be discussed in a later chapter.

What Time Does the Patient Wake up in the Morning?

Whilst everyone varies as to the time they normally wake up in the morning, some illnesses such as asthma or osteoarthritis generate early morning symptoms which may wake the patient early (Shapiro et al 1986, Monday et al 1987, Moldofsky 1987). Endogenous depression and unexplained insomnia are associated with early morning waking and many night wakings (Hartmann 1973, Borbély 1986).

Is the Patient Accustomed to a Sleep in the Daytime?

As already mentioned, the elderly may often take naps in the daytime, which can make up a high proportion of their total sleep time. However, there are other reasons why sleeping in the day may be an important part of an individual's customary sleep pattern. The British culture dictates on the whole that we have what is called a monophasic sleep pattern, sleep in one time span, usually at night (unless you are on night shift!). In countries with warm climates, the cultural tradition dictates biphasic sleep pattern, whereby the custom is to sleep in the afternoon, and then to go to bed much later at night for the second part of sleep. In the nursing assessment it should be identified whether the patient is used to a rest in the afternoon, whatever their cultural background, because young pre-school children as well as retired adults and the sick are often accustomed to it. As later chapters will demonstrate a rest in the afternoon can be positively beneficial for well-founded physiological reasons and should not therefore be discouraged in hospital unless for very well thought out reasons.

Drugs

Patients accustomed to taking night sedation will need to continue with it unless it is contra-indicated medically, because they may be dependent on it to sleep. Similarly patients who are used to taking analgesia at night for a painful condition will find it easier to go to sleep if they continue with this in hospital. Irwin (1989) found one of the predictive factors among medical patients as to whether they rated their sleep the same or better in hospital than at home, was that they had been given analgesia before going to sleep.

   Certain drugs can cause sleep disturbance (e.g. the older varieties of beta-blockers have been known to cause nightmares in some patients), whilst withdrawal of others can also have an effect (e.g. withdrawal from Diazepam can cause excessive dreaming and nightmares). The nurse should therefore be aware of any possible effects drug therapy may have on the patient and always have a reference source for drug information to hand.

Environmental Aspects of Assessment

For sleep onset to occur and for sleep quality to be good the environment must be conducive to it and therefore the nurse at night cannot divorce her assessment of the individual from the environment in which he is sleeping.

Auditory Awakening Thresholds

The auditory awakening threshold is the level of sound which will waken someone from sleep (Bonnet 1986). This threshold tends to decrease with age from 40 onwards, but the age-related differences are not as influential in determining responses as the individual differences in threshold (Zepelin et al 1984). In other words some people are particularly sensitive to noise and wake at the slightest sound, and others will sleep through anything. It is thought also that people are able to select noises to which they will wake (e.g. a mother will wake to the sound of her crying baby). Disturbance to sleep of any type, whether it be noise or some other form of discomfort, may not necessarily wake the person, but it will seriously interfere with the quality of their sleep. Therefore the nurse needs to be aware of any factors in the environment which could disrupt sleep and take action to neutralise their effect.

Noise

Much nursing research has shown that environmental factors are the main cause of sleep disturbance in hospital. Wilson-Barnett (1978) in a study of patients' feelings about their stay in hospital found that 36.2% of patients' nights in hospital had been disturbed, and that they felt unrested even though the disturbance to their sleep may not have been very long. Noise from other patients was blamed most frequently but noise and the lighting from the sluice or kitchen, if the patient's bed was in that vicinity, were also blamed. Patients in cubicles slept the best. Noisy equipment, such as steel bed-pans and basins, trollies, glass urinals, old-style commodes and ripple mattress motors, was identified as the main cause by Whitfield (1975) and again by Ogilvie (1980). The telephone ringing, doors banging, noisy footsteps and metal bins being emptied, nurses talking to other patients, and emergency admissions are other factors (Whitfield 1975, Wilson-Barnett 1978, Ogilvie 1980, Dodds 1980, Closs 1988).

The design of the ward can affect how noise is transmitted. Ogilvie (1980) showed that the noise levels in a modern 'race track' designed ward were significantly lower than they were in a Nightingale ward. Closs (1988) found that the design of ward was one of the key influences on the quality of surgical patients' sleep. There were significant differences between the sleep times of patients on the large Nightingale wards and those in the smaller areas. Those in the wards with bays reported total sleep times approximately one hour longer than those on Nightingale wards and they also reported fewer night wakings. In the light of these findings, Closs (1988) suggested that partitions should be erected in Nightingale wards to reduce the effect of noise.

Following on from this Irwin (1989) found there was no difference in the reported sleep times between medical patients on partitioned and non-partitioned Nightingale wards. It was suggested following this study that the key factor was management of the ward at night. Ogilvie (1980) had noted that organisation of the ward routine at night appeared to be directed towards staff convenience rather than patient care, because, on both wards in her study, the morning work commenced by bins being emptied at 05.30, thus disturbing most patients in the vicinity (Ogilvie 1980). Hicks (1990) studied the noise levels on wards before and after a quality assurance education programme for nurses involved in night duty regarding what created noise in the ward environment at night. Following the programme the noise levels in the wards were significantly quieter and patients slept longer, with fewer night wakings.

Lighting

The lighting needs to be dimmed for sleep onset to occur (Parkes 1985). The time at which lights go out in the ward needs to be well planned as part of the ward routine, but it should also allow for individuals to observe their own settling down time, and to go to sleep when they want to. The top lights can be dimmed quite early if it is complemented by the bed-side lights going on at the same time, and if prior thought has been paid to lighting areas required for nursing work. This creates a soft, calming light in the ward (however busy it may be) and allows each patient to settle at the time he chooses. Annoyance from lights in areas such as the sluice or kitchen should be considered and prevented; and window blinds or curtains drawn to prevent interference from light from outside the ward.

Ambient temperature

The ward temperature should be comfortable in order for sleep onset to occur and for sleep to remain undisturbed. Closs (1988) found that this was an important factor patients said disturbed them. It has been demonstrated that extremes of temperature will affect the sleep cycle and result in restless sleep and many awakenings (Parkes 1985, Karacan et al 1978).

Mattress

Hard surfaces are difficult to sleep on. Over 50% of the patients in the Closs (1988) study had the old type of horse-hair mattress and they rated their sleep very badly. German studies (Parkes 1985), proved that subjects spent more time in the transitional phase of sleep (which is not considered to be sleep at all by some authorities) if they were on a hard surface. Patients in pain will find a hard mattress particularly difficult to sleep on. The nurse therefore needs to include in her assessment how comfortable the patient seems to be on the hospital bed and relate this to the pressure area assessment and pressure relieving measures.

Evaluation of Nursing Care and Patient Progress During the Night

'Evaluation' in the Cambridge English Dictionary means to 'state the value of'. In the nursing process it is to state the value of the problems identified and the effects of the nursing interventions planned for them. It may be to elaborate on problems already identified, highlight new problems, and to suggest new interventions for problems that have not resolved. It is therefore an important part of further diagnosis, planning and intervention, and should be carried out at regular pre-planned intervals. It should also be continuous so that intelligent use can be made of new information as it becomes known.

In the case of the patient at night, it is here that the role of the night nurse is of particular value. It can be of greater value if the information she collects is done in a systematic way, which can be easily interpreted and used by her colleagues in the day to act upon appropriately.

Sleep

The research findings regarding nursing evaluation of patients' sleep are very disappointing. Dodds (1980) found patients reported minimal contact with nurses during the night. What there was, was normally linked to nursing care. Over half the respondents felt that the nurses were unaware of their difficulties sleeping, and this was supported by the fact that one third of the nursing reports were found to be at variance with what the patients said about their sleep. Closs (1988) found that the evaluation notes frequently had only a cursory mention of the patient's sleep pattern. Cohen (1983), in a study of elderly institutionalised patients in America, found that the ratings of patients' sleep on a five point scale by nurses and patients did not correlate and that nurses had failed to identify problem sleepers.

The evaluation of patients' sleep at night is not easy if there are no specific and consistent indices for everyone to use and communicate with. There is therefore a need for nurses to use a consistent approach in evaluation, such as the one used in the earlier assessment.

Because what people say about their sleep correlates so well with their sleep EEG in sleep studies, it would seem that in nursing what patients say about their sleep pattern should be included as an important part of the evaluation of their sleep. This is more likely to have validity than anything the nurse has observed. People have their eyes closed in all stages of the sleep cycle, and only an EEG will be able to determine what stage of sleep they are in, not an observer by the bed-side. If the framework of the instrument already discussed is used, nurses will soon be able to identify the different types of sleep problem their patient has. For example:

> The patient may have taken a long time to go to sleep (had a long *sleep onset latency*); he may have had several *night awakenings* for a specific reason; his *morning waking time* might not yet have arrived because the symptoms which had kept him awake in the night have resolved, and it will be appropriate for the day staff to let him wake up later in his own time.

Sometimes patients will report that their sleep was uninterrupted but that they do not feel refreshed in the morning. As the following chapter on physiology will clarify, anything which interferes with the normal sleep pattern may have this effect; but certain sedative drugs and alcohol may induce an abnormal type of sleep which does not refresh the person, because the important parts of the sleep cycle have been depressed. In this situation, the patient may wake after a night of awakenings feeling drowsy, irritable and unrested. A change of medication may improve the situation, but sleep disturbance of this type can also be associated with certain illnesses, including endogenous depression, so records of subjective feelings after sleep are important to enable appropriate observation, evaluation and care planning by the whole nursing team.

Factors Which Might Affect Patients' Sleep in Hospital

Length of Time in Hospital

People find it difficult to sleep in a strange environment, but they adapt over time. Patients also seem to adapt to being in hospital. Over half the patients in the Wilson-Barnett (1978) study said they had more disturbed nights at the beginning of their stay in hospital than towards the end of their stay. Dodds (1980) also found that the number of days since admission was a factor in patients sleeping better, possibly because they had become accustomed to the hospital environment and ward routine. Most sleep surveys of patients in hospital exclude those whose first night it is, because of the possibility that their sleep will be disturbed by the strange surroundings.

The Effects of Post-Surgical Stress

Closs (1988) found no association between days since admission and improved sleep times, but this may have been due to the fact that all the patients in the study were surgical patients and many other factors such as post-surgical stress can be present for some days. Post-surgical stress, together with the effects of the drugs used for anaesthesia and post-operative analgesia, have been shown to disrupt sleep patterns for some time after the event (Aurell and Elmquist 1985, Kavey and Altshuler 1979, Lehmkuhl et al 1987). Therefore a calm, sleep inducing environment on surgical wards may be more important than in other areas as there is more to overcome in relation to the patient's stress levels.

Night Signs and Symptoms

The nurse at night is in the best position to observe the patient sleeping and identify what symptoms cause discomfort and sleep disturbance. Some of the symptoms and pathologies involved are included below:

Snoring	Indigestion
Restlessness	Pain
Nightmares	Anxiety
Dyspnoea	Depression
Palpitations	Confusion
Nocturia	Insomnia
Enuresis/incontinence	

The aetiology and nursing interventions for many of these will be discussed in later chapters. Suffice it to say here that the role of the nurse at night in observing, assessing and evaluating the presence and progress of them should play an important role in the overall assessment and evaluation of the patient's total care.

Effects in the Day of Sleep Deprivation

As the patient requires coherent, continuous care throughout the 24 hours of the day, his management should be guided by information gathered at all times in the nursing cycle. The nurse at night must contribute to the assessment, evaluation and management of patient care in the day, and the nurse during the day should be able to contribute information to the assessment and evaluation of the patient's sleep and night-time problems.

The nurses in the daytime are in the best position in diagnose the incipient symptoms of sleep deprivation:

Daytime sleepiness
Frequent yawning
Listlessness
Lethargy
Ptosis (drooping eyelids)
Nystagmus (oscillatory movements of the eyeballs)
Red conjunctiva and 'whites of the eyes'
Dark circles under the eyes
Irritability

During the day evidence of a problem with sleeping may be manifest by any of the signs and symptoms above, as well as patient complaints following admission that they have difficulty falling asleep, staying asleep, or that they do not feel well rested. Patients at this time may ask for night sedation as a temporary measure to enable them to sleep in hospital (Kemp 1984). If they have had a good initial assessment, the nurse will know if this is a hospital-induced problem. If the patient is questioned in a methodical way using the framework of the observable features of sleep already described, then some sense can be made of his complaints. It is important to establish the cause of lack of sleep, so that if possible nursing actions can pre-empt what should be the last resort – night sedation.

Conclusion

The effective nursing management of any patient relies on a good assessment founded on a sound nursing knowledge base. The traditional role of the night nurse has been that of 'caretaker', rather than a partner in the team giving 24-hour care. This has had implications for the contributions of night staff to patient assessment and evaluation in the past. As later chapters will show, sleep is far too important a part of the patient's well-being for this state of affairs to continue. Nurses at night see the patient at his most vulnerable. His sleep or the lack of it can seriously affect the way he may cope with his illness. It is time for nurses during the night to be aware of the importance of their role in the entirety of patient management, and for those in the day-time to enable contributions about night-time problems to be incorporated in the overall assessment, evaluation and management of patient care.

Florence Nightingale seemed to understand far better than nurses in the twentieth century the importance of sleep. Sleep research is proving her right. If as nurses we have failed in the past to enable patients to sleep as we should, the methods of the sleep scientists are now showing us the way. We should not be too proud to use the methods they have found valid and reliable to assess and evaluate patients' sleep. In doing so, our understanding and communication of patients' problems at night can only improve, and our actions to resolve them become more effective.

References

Aurell J and Elmquist M (1985) Sleep in the surgical intensive care unit: continuous polygraphic recording of sleep in 9 patients receiving post-operative care. *British Medical Journal*, **290**, 1029–1032.

Beszterczey A (1977) Insomnia in cancer patients. *Canadian Medical Association Journal*, **116**, 355.

Bixler E O and Vela-Bueno A (1987) Normal sleep: patterns and mechanisms. *Seminars in Neurology*, **7**, 3, 227–235.

Bonnet M H (1986) Auditory thresholds during continuing sleep. *Biological Psychology*, **22**, 3–10.

Borbély A (1986) *Secrets of Sleep*. London: Penguin.

Brezinova V and Oswald I (1972) Sleep after a bed-time drink. *British Medical Journal*, **5811**, 2, 431–433.

Carpenito L J (1989) *Nursing Diagnosis: Application to Clinical Practice* (3rd edn) Philadelphia: J B Lippincott.

Carskadon M A, Dement W C, Mitler M M, Guillemniault C N, Zarcone V P and Spiegel (1976) Self-reports versus sleep laboratory findings in 122 drug-free subjects with complaints of chronic insomnia. *American Journal of Psychiatry*, **133**, 12, 1382–1388.

Carter D (1984) *Sleeping Soundly? Sleep and the Low-Dependency Hospital Patient.* Unpublished MSc thesis. University of Glasgow.

Closs S J (1988) *A Nursing Study of Sleep on Surgical Wards*. Report for the Scottish Home and Health Dept. University of Edinburgh.

Cohen D, Eisdorfer C, Prinz P, Breen A, Davis M and Gadsby A (1983) Sleep disturbances in the institutionalized aged. *American Geriatrics Society*, **31**, 79–83.

Dodds E J (1980) *Slept Well? A Study of Ward Activity and Nurse Patient Interaction at Night*. Unpublished MSc thesis. University of Surrey.

Frankel B L, Coursey R D, Buchbinder R and Synder F (1976) Recorded and reported sleep in chronic and primary insomnia. *Archives of General Psychiatry*, **33**, 615–623.

Hartmann J (1973) *The Functions of Sleep*. London: Yale University Press.

Hayter J (1983) Sleep behaviours in older persons. *Nursing Research*, **32**, 4, 242–246.

Hicks F M (1990) *An Evaluation of Outcome Measures Following Standard Setting for Noise Levels on Wards at Night*. Unpublished BSc Dissertation. University of Surrey.

Horne J A (1988) *Why We Sleep: The Functions of Sleep in Humans and Other Mammals*. Oxford: Oxford University Press.

Horne J A and Ostberg O (1976) A self-assessment questionnaire to determine morningness and eveningness in human circadian rhythms. *International Journal of Chronobiology*, **4**, 97–110.

Hunt J M and Marks-Maran D J (1986) *Nursing Care Plans: the Nursing Process at Work* (2nd edn) Chichester: John Wiley.

Irwin H P (1989) *A Comparative Study of the Self-Reported Sleep Patterns of Medical Patients on Nightingale Wards With and Without Partitions.* Unpublished MSc dissertation. University of Manchester.

Johns M W (1977) Validity of subjective reports of sleep latency in normal subjects. *Ergonomics*, **20**, 6, 683–690.

Johns M W and Doré C (1978) Sleep at home and in the sleep laboratory: disturbance by recording procedures. *Ergonomics*, **21**, 5, 325–330.

Johnson J E (1986) Sleep and bed-time routines of non-institutionalised aged women. *Journal Community Health Nursing*, **3**, 117–125.

Karacan I, Thornby J I, Anch A M and Williams R L (1978) The effects of high ambient temperature on the sleep of young men. *Sleep Research*, **7**, 171.

Kavey N B and Altshuler K Z (1979) Sleep in herniorraphy patients. *American Journal of Surgery*. **138**, 682–687.

Kemp J (1984) Nursing at night. *Journal of Advanced Nursing*, **9**, 217–223.

Korner E, Bertha G, Flooh E, Reinhart B, Wolf R and Lechner H (1986) Sleep inducing effects of L-tryptophan. *European Neurology*, **25**, 2, 75–81.

Lehmkuhl P, Prass D and Pichlmayr I (1987) General anaesthesia and postnarcotic sleep disorders. *Neuropsychobiology*, **18**, 37–42.

Moldofsky H (1986) Sleep and musculoskeletal pain. *American Journal of Medicine*, **81** (Suppl. 3A), 85–89.

Moldofsky H, Lue F A and Saskin P (1987) Sleep and morning pain in primary osteoarthritis. *Journal of Rheumatology*, **14**, 124–128.

Monday J, Montplaisir J and Malo J L (1987) Dream process in asthmatic subjects with nocturnal attacks. *American Journal of Psychiatry*, **144**, 5, 638–640.

Morgan K (1987) *Sleep and Aging*. London: Croom Helm.

Murphy F, Bentley S, Ellis B W and Dudley H (1977) Sleep deprivation in patients undergoing operation: a factor in the stress of surgery. *British Medical Journal*, **2**, 1521–1522.

Murray J, Dunn G, Wiliams P and Tarnapolsky A (1981) Factors affecting the consumption of psychotrophic drugs. *Psychological Medicine*, **11**, 551–560.

Nightingale F (1859) *Notes on Nursing: what it is, and what it is not.* Edinburgh: Churchill Livingstone (1980).

Ogilvie J A (1980) Sources and levels of noise on the ward at night. *Nursing Times*, 31 July, 1363–1366.

Parkes J D (1985) *Sleep and its Disorders*. Philadelphia: W B Saunders.

Sewitch D E (1984) The perceptual uncertainty of having slept. *Psychophysiology*, **21**, 3, 243–259.

Shapiro C M, Catterall J R, Montgomery I, Raab G M, Douglas N J (1986) Do asthmatics suffer bronchoconstriction during rapid eye movement sleep? *British Medical Journal*, **292**, 3rd May, 1161–1164.

Webb W W (1982) Sleep in older persons: sleep structures of 50–60-year-old men and women. *Journal of Gerontology*, **37**, 5, 581–586.

Whitfield S (1975) Noise on the ward at night. *Nursing Times*, 13 March, 408–412.

Wilson-Barnett J (1978) In hospital: patients' feelings and opinions. *Nursing Times Occasional Papers*, **74**, 8 29–32.

Wilson-Barnett J and Carrigy A (1978) Factors influencing patients' emotional reactions to hospitalization. *Journal of Advanced Nursing*, **3**, 221–229.

Zepelin H, Mcdonald C S and Zammit G K (1984) Effects of age on auditory awakening thresholds. *Journal of Gerontology*, **39**, 3, 294–300.

Chapter 3
The Physiology
of Sleep
Penny Irwin

Introduction

For centuries sleep has mystified those who have studied it. From classical times there have been attempts to explain it. The ancient Greeks associated it with foretelling the future through dreams and with healing. The sick made pilgrimages to sleep in certain temples in the hope that a god would appear to them in their dreams and that they would be healed (Empson 1989). In more modern times sleep has come to be regarded as a 'passive' state, which can be interrupted at will (Kemp 1984). This is possibly because of some of the traditional beliefs about the physiology of sleep. However, sleep research is beginning to demonstrate that sleep is an 'active' process, brought about by the activation of various structures in the brain (Borbély 1986). In this state many phenomena occur which are vital to the continued health and well-being of the individual.

This chapter will examine the pattern of sleep and some of the methods used to study it; different theories about the control and function of sleep; sleep disturbance and the effects of sleep deprivation; and finally different aspects of abnormal sleep, including the more common sleep disorders, and the effects different illnesses have on sleep.

The Methods of Sleep Research

The problem for nurses who are trying to find out about sleep is that it is a very wide field of research. The *Annual Bibliography of Sleep Research* published by the Brain Research Institute lists over a thousand articles each year for the 1980s. The disciplines involved in the study of sleep include neuroscientists, paediatricians, psychiatrists, pharmacologists, engineers, animal behaviourists, physiologists, psychologists and biochemists (Webb 1983). Much of this work is therefore extremely esoteric and complex. However, research is progressing at such a rapid rate and the discoveries becoming so important that nurses can no longer be left in ignorance without some attempt to translate the complexities of this multi-disciplinary research into a form whereby it can be used to enhance the care of patients. The aim of this chapter is to do that.

In the 1920s it was discovered that the electrical activity of the brain could be visualised on the electro-encephalogram (EEG). It became evident that the EEG during sleep differed from that obtained during wakefulness, as it showed a distinct pattern with well-defined stages, occurring in a cycle. Subsequently it has been shown that there are also changes in muscle tone which can be measured by electromyogram (EMG). In 1952 two researchers, Azerinsky and Kleitman, discovered that one particular stage of sleep on the EEG was associated with rapid eye movements, which can be measured by electro-oculogram (EOG).

When sleep is studied, it is usually carried out with normal subjects in sleep laboratories especially designed for the purpose. Electrodes are placed on the subject's scalp for EEG, chin for EMG and temple for EOG (this form of measurement is given the name polysomnography). The subject then settles for the night with all these electrodes in place in a quiet room. It has been found, not surprisingly, that the presence of the electrodes can disturb subjects' sleep pattern (Johns et al 1978), but that they become accustomed to the strange environment and sleep paraphernalia after one or two nights in the laboratory. 'The first night effect' as it is called is usually taken into account in the design of studies in the laboratory, and the first night's recordings are not used in the final study results (Horne 1988a).

When the subjects in the sleep laboratory wake in the morning it is usual for them to be interviewed about their sleep that night using the observable features of sleep described in the previous chapter, i.e. their settling time, their sleep onset time, how many awakenings they had and the reasons for them, and morning waking time. They may also be asked about how refreshed or drowsy they feel, depending on the nature and purpose of the research study in progress.

The analysis of the print-outs from all the recordings is carried out in conjunction with the interview results. In recent years, power spectrum analysis of EEG results has enabled researchers to look very much more closely at subtle differences in the frequency and amplitude of the EEG signal, and shown that the power of the signal as well as its pattern is related to the quality of the sleep being studied. This is leading to significant discoveries about the differences in the quality of sleep (Borbély 1986; Astrom et al 1989).

Much of the knowledge gained about sleep in hospital and sleep in various illnesses has been gained using polysomnographic techniques on hospitalised patients. However, because of the complexity of the equipment and the disturbance to the individual undergoing the study polysomnography is not appropriate in all sleep research. Because the responses to interview in normal subjects involved in sleep studies correlate well with their polysomnographic data (Johns 1977, Johns et al 1978), it is considered valid in research where knowledge of the specific sleep stages is not required not to use polysomnography, but to interview the patient using the observable features of sleep and other qualitative measures in the questionnaire (Dodds 1980, Carter

1984, Closs 1988, Ellis et al 1981, Irwin 1989). Other techniques related to the purpose of the study, such as observation or the use of acoustic equipment may also be used concurrently.

The Pattern of Normal Sleep

Traditionally, the sleep cycle has been described in the light of the particular characteristics it shows in polysomnography. This indicates that there are five distinct stages of the sleep cycle, which are named according to whether or not they are associated with rapid eye movements (REM) (Azerinsky and Kleitman 1953). These stages normally occur in the following sequence during the course of a night's sleep and are described in Figure 3.1.

1. Stage 1 Non-REM (NREM) Sleep is a phase which occurs at sleep onset. The EEG shows small, irregular (theta) waves, whilst there are rolling eye movements and the muscle tone is tense. This phase lasts from 30 seconds to 7 minutes in normal young adults and does not normally reappear during the subsequent sleep cycles (Borbély 1986). This can vary with age, illness and disturbance from outside stimuli. It is the view of most authorities that stage 1 sleep is only a transition phase from wakefulness to sleep and does not constitute part of true sleep (Horne 1988a, page 9).

2. Stage 2 NREM Sleep follows stage 1 sleep and makes up 45% of total

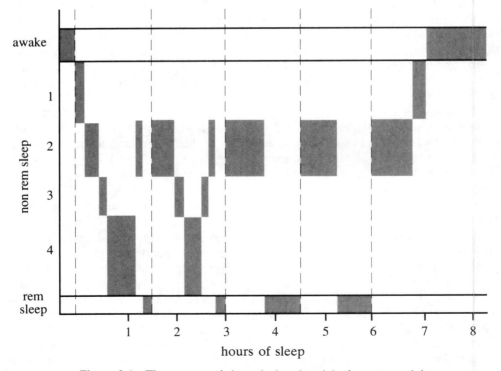

Figure 3.1 The pattern of sleep during the night for young adults

sleep (Horne 1988a). The EEG is characterised by larger waves than stage 1 sleep, with rapid bursts of sleep spindles and occasional large slow waves (K-complexes). EOG shows the eyes to be still and EMG that the muscle tension is reduced. Stage 2 is counted by sleep scientists as the onset of true sleep (Horne 1988a, p 9). In the first cycle of the night it lasts a few minutes, but during a night's sleep stage 2 constitutes an increasing proportion of each cycle, and is the beginning of each subsequent sleep cycle (Borbély 1986).

3. **Stage 3 NREM Sleep** is characterised by 20% to 50% delta waves on EEG, low muscle tone on EMG, and the eyes are still on the EOG. It follows stage 2 NREM in the sleep cycle and constitutes the start of Slow Wave Sleep (SWS) (sometimes called Deep sleep, or Delta sleep) (Borbély 1986, Horne 1988a).

4. **Stage 4 NREM Sleep** follows stage 3, making up the remainder of SWS. It is characterised by over 50% delta waves on EEG, no eye movements, and low muscle tension. It lasts thirty to forty minutes in the first sleep cycle, and is halved in the second. SWS does not reappear in the sleep cycles in the latter part of the night. Blood pressure is low, heart rate is reduced and breathing regular. The auditory awakening threshold is the highest in this sleep stage. In normal young adults SWS is said to make up 13% of total sleep (Horne 1988a).

Body movements occur naturally during sleep, usually at the end of a period of SWS (Borbély 1986).

SWS has attracted much attention in recent years as it coincides with certain important physiological events. The largest surge of Human Growth Hormone of the day occurs with the onset of SWS. This seems to occur only in the first sleep cycle. Children with short stature are often found to have poor SWS and to be growth hormone deficient. Young adults who are growth hormone deficient have been shown to have decreased SWS (Astrom 1990). Stress of any type can interfere with the normal sleep cycle and mean that SWS is not attained. Recurrent depression is associated with less SWS and reduced growth hormone secretion (Jarrett et al 1990).

Moldofsky et al (1986a) have shown that SWS is also associated with dramatic changes in the activity of some immune factors, in particular Interleukin–1.

5. **REM Sleep** SWS is followed by a short period of stage 2 NREM sleep before the appearance of Rapid Eye Movement (REM) sleep. REM sleep is associated with rapid eye movements, total muscle relaxation (to the point of paralysis of motor muscles), irregular breathing, and surges in blood pressure and heart rate. REM sleep lasts only a few minutes in the first sleep cycle but increases in amount with each cycle, until by the morning a substantial proportion of the sleep is REM sleep. After each period of REM sleep, a new sleep cycle begins with Stage 2 sleep. Each sleep cycle lasts approximately 90 minutes.

REM sleep is renowned for the fact that dreams can be recalled on awakening from it. It has been proven that dreaming occurs in all stages of the sleep cycle, but that those in REM sleep are often more vivid, particularly later in

the night, than those in the other sleep stages (Borbély 1986, Parkes 1985).
It is thought that REM sleep might provide the means of coping with stressful
situations, and also to be involved in information processing and the consoli-
dation of learning (Smith and Kelly 1988, Wright and Koulack 1987). It has
been shown that the other stages of the sleep cycle may be involved in
consolidating learning (Ambrosini 1988) but not to the same extent as REM
sleep. In the 1960s and 1970s REM sleep was considered the most important
phase of the sleep cycle, but in recent years discoveries about the rather
ignominiously named NREM stages of sleep, in particular Stages 3 and 4,
have shown that the entirety of the sleep cycle is important.

Normal Variations in Sleep Pattern

The pattern of sleep changes throughout life. Premature babies sleep most
of the time and 80% of their sleep is REM sleep. This falls to 60% at 36
weeks gestation, and to 50% at term. Babies up until they are 4 months old
have REM sleep from sleep onset, but from the time they are 4 months old
they enter sleep through NREM in the adult pattern. Total sleep time
decreases as childhood progresses and the proportion of REM sleep becomes
less, falling from 50% to 30%. The high proportion of REM sleep in the
young has led some to suggest that it is important for brain growth and
development in some way (Parkes 1985).

Young and middle aged adults mainly have the sleep pattern described in
Figure 3.1 and Table 3.1, but this may vary between individuals depending
on local, cultural and personal factors. Most people sleep between 7 and 8
hours a night. However, there are variations from 5.5 to 9.5 hours and much
research has been directed at the differences between long and short sleepers
(Borbély 1986, Horne 1988a). The long sleepers seem to have the same
amount of SWS as short sleepers, but a lot more REM and stage 2 sleep.

Table 3.1 Percentage of a night's sleep spent in each sleep stage by a young adult (from Horne J (1988a) Why we sleep: The functions of sleep in humans and other mammals)

Stage	Percentage
Stage 1	5%
Stage 2	45%
Stage 3	7%
Stage 4	13%
REM sleep	30%

REM sleep seems to remain fairly constant from puberty onwards (Parkes
1985). As age advances, people have increased difficulty getting off to sleep,
and once asleep, they may be subject to increasingly frequent and prolonged
awakenings, and shorter sleep stages. This pattern is evident in 50–60 year
olds (Webb 1982). The elderly are more likely to be awoken by noise (Zepelin

1984), for frequent toileting requirements, and because they feel stiff and uncomfortable because reduced mobility has prevented them from taking the natural movements that occur in sleep. They will often take day-time naps as a part of their regular sleep pattern (Hayter 1983, Morgan 1987). This may result in them waking in the early hours of the morning (Horne 1988a).

There is a difference between the quality of sleep of men and women in all stages of life. Men do not sleep as well as women, possibly due to the penile tumescence which occurs during REM sleep. Consistent results from studies into the quality of their sleep prove women, even in old age, sleep better (Webb 1982, Horne 1988a, Reynolds 1986).

The Control of Sleep

There have been many theories about the control of sleep. Most have rested on the existence of a sleep centre. Arguments from the different schools of thought have persisted through the years, until it is now thought to be controlled by several interlinked centres in the brain, several neurotransmitters or sleep substances, the amount of preceding time awake and the body's 24-hour 'clock' (the circadian rhythms). Ultimately many factors influence sleep onset and its maintenance. The physiological centres and substances interact with each other, with the environment, with the individual's lifestyle, and with the bodily and the mental state to control it.

The most well-known 'centre' in the brain to be involved in sleep is the reticular formation, a complex of nerve cells and fibres stretching throughout the brain stem, with connections to the spinal cord, cerebellum, cranial nerve nuclei and forebrain. It is associated mainly with arousal. The feed-back loop theory of wakefulness suggests that the reticular formation keeps the body awake by responding to all the many sensory stimuli transported along the pathways from all over the body. Sleep, by this theory, occurs when at the end of the day fewer pathways send messages because of fatigue and, as sensory input declines, sleep occurs. Research shows that noise, hard surfaces, unpleasant ambient temperature and pain lead to poor quality sleep (Parkes 1985, Closs 1988), so the reticular formation most certainly has a role in disturbing the sleep pattern by maintaining a level of arousal in response to stimuli, but it does not actively induce sleep.

This rather passive view of how sleep occurs is now only held to be part of the control of sleep. The centres thought to control sleep in a more active sense include the raphe nucleus, thalamus and basal forebrain. There is still argument over the exact function of the all these centres, but it is thought that they become activated to induce sleep, or certain types of sleep, rather than being passive as in the feed-back loop theory (Bixler et al 1987). How these centres are activated is still a cause for conjecture but it is looking increasingly as if a variety of neurotransmitters may be involved.

In recent years there has been a revival of interest in the theory that there is a sleep substance. Aristotle thought that vapours rose to the head following a meal and overwhelmed the consciousness, resulting in sleep. Researchers in the late nineteenth and early twentieth centuries hypothesised that various substances called hypnotoxins built up in the blood resulting in sleep (Parkes 1985, Borbély 1986, Horne 1988a). These were called humoral theories and for the most part of this century were regarded as being of little significance by those in the mainstream of sleep research.

In the 1960s, a substance was discovered in the cerebrospinal fluid of sleep deprived animals, which when injected into others made them sleep longer than their controls. This was named Factor 'S' (Borbély 1986). By the 1980s, refinements had occurred and other substances had been found and synthesised, which are being currently tested all over the world (Horne 1988b). They include Delta sleep inducing peptide (DSIP), Prostaglandin D2, Serotonin, sleep promoting substance (SPS), and muramyl dipeptide.

Muramyl dipeptide (MDP) is a compound that is derived from muramic acid, which is one of the 5 basic amino acids which make up Factor 'S'. It has been found to have important sleep-inducing effects, but it is also an important immuno-regulator which triggers the production of Interleukin-1 (IL-1). It also increases body temperature (Kreuger 1986). Both MDP and IL-1 have been found to induce SWS (Kreuger 1984), which is perhaps an indicator of the importance of this phase of sleep in the body's response to illness. Most researchers, are very cautious about making extravagant claims for this discovery. They say that it is not possible to say at present if MDPs or IL-1 are involved in the regulation of normal sleep, but admit that they could be the reason why people feel so sleepy when they have an infection (Kreuger 1986).

It may be that different centres and different substances control different phases of the sleep cycle. The sleep-wake cycle is linked to the body's biological internal 'clock', the circadian rhythms (circa = about, dies = day). It is thought at present that there may be two or more such 'clocks', one that regulates the rhythm of NREM sleep, and another that regulates physiological functions such as body temperature, the secretion of various hormones, electrolyte balance and REM sleep (Dijk et al 1989, Moore-Ede 1983, Horne 1988a). Circadian rhythms are more or less in unison with the 24-hour day/ night cycle but need to be kept in tune with environmental time by 'Zeitgebers' (time-givers), which are regular daily environmental events such as alarm clocks, meal times or going to work.

Normally sleep-wake cycles are in tune with the circadian rhythms, but if this harmony is desynchronised by a changed pattern of existence, the subject may feel lethargic and 'out of sorts', as in jet-lag or shift work (Borbély 1986, Horne 1988a). Seasonal changes in daylight time also affect circadian rhythm. It has been demonstrated that human beings exposed to bright light early in the morning shift their circadian rhythms (measured by the advance in time of the rise in plasma melatonin secretion in the evenings, as well as an advance in the time of the rise in body temperature during sleep), and subsequently sleep for a shorter time quite spontaneously, without any ill effects. When this happens it is at the expense of morning REM sleep, and NREM sleep is unaffected (Dijk et al 1989).

Coming into hospital can alter the patient's routine considerably, especially at night when bed-times and morning waking times may be different to the habitual ones at home. The times when people go to bed and get up are very individual. Horne and Ostberg (1976) found two distinct types of people, those who went to bed early and got up early ('morning' types), and those who preferred to stay up late at night and 'lie in' in the morning ('evening' types). They accounted for these variations as being a manifestation of individual variations in circadian rhythms. The rigid routines found in hospital were criticised in the National Health Service Management Consultancy Service Report on the Night Nursing Services (1987), and nursing studies into patients' sleep in hospital demonstrate that routines can result in altered and disturbed sleep patterns (Carter 1984, Closs 1988, Dodds 1980), with greater sleep onset latencies due to altered bed-times, and a feeling of being sleep-deprived when woken early in the morning.

The number of day-time naps has been found to increase in normal subjects confined to bed rest for several days in an environment without time cues (Campbell 1984), so in the less active environment that hospital is for some people, with time cues that are different or relatively unimportant, some may 'nap' more in the day-time, which may also affect their sleep at night. Moldofsky et al (1986a) found that in afternoon 'naps' where SWS occurred there were, as in night-time SWS, increases in immunological activity. Therefore, rest in the afternoons can be beneficial, especially if it is making up for lost sleep at night.

Theories on the Function of Sleep

There have been many theories on the function of sleep over the years but in essence there are two main schools of thought: the Behaviourist school and the Restorative school (Webb 1983).

Behaviourists, at the most extreme, regard sleep as an 'instinct' (Meddis 1983) which during evolution enabled animals to remain still, away from predators; and which enables human beings to remain quiet when there is nothing much to do, as at night, or in hot countries during the hottest part of the day.

The Restorative school by contrast believe that sleep is a time of body restitution (Hartmann 1973, Adam 1980, Adam and Oswald 1977). They point especially to such factors as the release of Human Growth Hormone during Slow Wave Sleep (SWS) and the apparent high rate of mitosis that occurs during sleep (Adam and Oswald 1977). Horne (1983) argues that there is no proof of the immediate action of Human Growth Hormone released during sleep increasing mitosis in human beings. He says that it is possible that the high level of HGH during sleep could be a protective mechanism against protein breakdown during the night fast.

Most nurses will have a natural affinity with the restorative theories, having seen patients well rested and improved following a good night's sleep. However, it is important to understand that the two theories have an equal contribution to make to our understanding of the complex and universal phenomenon of sleep.

The predominant view amongst sleep theorists and researchers now points to the first few hours of sleep as the most essential for health and well-being (Borbély 1986, Oswald 1980, Horne 1988a). Horne (1988a) differentiates between 'core' (or obligatory) sleep, the restorative part, which constitutes the first few hours of sleep, when SWS and some REM sleep occurs; and 'optional' (or facultative) sleep, which comes in the latter part of the night, its function being mainly comfort and relaxation. People will vary in their need for optional sleep, but everyone needs at least 5 hours containing the crucial components of core sleep. The main reason that SWS and some REM sleep are believed to be so important is that research into sleep deprivation shows that all of SWS and some of REM sleep is made up during the recovery sleep following deprivation, pointing to some essential function of this part of the sleep cycle. Horne (1988a) believes this function to be brain restitution, as it is the Central Nervous System (CNS) that appears to be so deleteriously affected by sleep deprivation (as shown by poor performance of mental exercises) and that revives following recovery sleep.

Other functions for sleep remain a matter for debate. Researchers have shown that Interleukin–1 increases SWS (Kreuger et al 1984). At present they are tentative in making definitive statements about the exact relationship of SWS to the immune system. Most indicate that it is too soon to say that SWS deprivation will depress the immune response, but they do point out the adverse effect that stress has on the sleep cycle and that stress is also known to depress the immune response (Horne 1988a, Moldofsky et al 1986a). They indicate that a combination of stress and sleep deprivation would depress the immune response, which is likely to be the case with acutely ill patients in hospital. In a few more years no doubt, many of these questions will be answered, but in the meantime nurses should take into account the importance of the first few hours of sleep for patients.

Sleep Onset and Maintenance

For sleep to occur it is important that there is an absence of sensory stimuli, for example, that there is quiet, that the lights are dim and the ambient temperature pleasant. A comfortable bed is very important, both in helping sleep onset to occur and in the maintenance of sleep. Studies quoted by Parkes (1985) showed that hard surfaces caused more body movements, more awakenings and more stage 1 sleep than softer surfaces.

Delay in sleep onset is called sleep onset latency. The more common reasons for sleep onset latency in hospital patients is the unfamiliar environment, the surrounding activity and noise, anxiety, pain and discomfort associated with their condition (Phillips and Cousins 1986) and missing loved ones.

Sleep Disturbance

Noise can disturb the sleeper in different ways. People vary in how sensitive they are to noise. Some have been found to waken at a threshold of 15dB(A) and others at 100dB(A). The elderly awaken more readily to noise than younger people. Auditory awakening thresholds are lowest in stage 1 and highest in stage 4, being variable in REM (Parkes 1985, p 47). They are thought to be lower for meaningful stimuli, like the cry of a baby to its mother, or someone calling the person's name. Research suggests that the brain still processes auditory information during sleep, particularly in stages 1 and 2 (Bonnet 1986a).

Noise may not wake the subject, but they will shift to a lighter phase of sleep, usually stage 1 NREM (Bonnet 1986a), which as has already been mentioned is not considered to be true sleep at all. If the disturbance is frequent, this makes it impossible for the person to maintain or even achieve SWS, or REM sleep. All these stages of sleep are particularly 'fragile' and may not occur if there is disturbance, danger or distress. This has been shown to happen in polysomnographic studies of patients on intensive care units, recovery units and general wards following surgery (Hilton 1976, Kavey and Altshuler 1979, Orr and Stahl 1977), where many were found to spend most of the night in stage 1 sleep.

Other disturbing factors have the same effect. Enuresis is known to occur normally in the first third of the night, just after the first period of SWS, and it has been shown that the subject left in a wet bed will not return to the normal sleep cycle, including the second wave of SWS, whilst the subject who has his bed changed does so (Williams 1971). Pain will also have the same effect.

The Effects of Sleep Deprivation

Sleep deprivation can be described in four ways:

1. **Total** – when the individual has no sleep over a span of time outside the normal sleep–wake period. This usually applies to being awake for a period over several days.
2. **Partial** – when for some reason the full amount of sleep that an individual normally has is not obtained. This is the usual type seen in hospital.
3. **REM** – when REM sleep is missing from the sleep cycle. In hospital one of the most likely reasons for this will be drugs that suppress REM sleep, e.g. barbiturates, phenothiazines, Mono-amine-oxidase inhibitors, amphetamines, narcotics, alcohol and benzodiazepines (Fass 1971, Manfredi and Kales 1987).
4. **SWS** – when SWS sleep is missing from the sleep cycle. Certain drugs can also suppress SWS, e.g. alcohol, barbiturates, higher doses of Diazepam, chloral hydrate (Fass 1971, Manfredi and Kales 1987).

The main effects of total sleep deprivation are on the central nervous system, in particular the brain, so the most common symptoms are speech slurring; memory lapses (including disorientation with time); reduced ability to perform psychomotor skills accurately, particularly if these are of a monotonous nature; and irritability. The body temperature falls by 1 degree centigrade, so the subject feels cold. There are visual misperceptions (not hallucinations), especially after prolonged deprivation, such as 5 days or more (Horne 1988a).

Partial deprivation may result in some of these symptoms, as most nurses after night duty know only too well.

The physiological effects of sleep deprivation seem to be relatively minor compared to the psychomotor effects. Various studies into such indices as urinary cortisols, blood sedimentation rates, urinary catecholamine levels, heart rate and blood pressure showed no significant changes associated with sleep deprivation (Horne 1988a).

Some have argued that lack of SWS will have adverse effects on how people feel and perform the following day (Agnew et al 1967, Frankel et al 1976). It has recently been shown that subjective feelings of sleepiness and performance loss are no more likely to be present in those with selective SWS deprivation than those who have had their sleep disturbed at set intervals (Bonnet 1986b). It was concluded in this study that it was the periodicity and frequency of the disruption which was the determining factor in performance loss and subjective sleepiness, possibly because of the fragmentation of SWS. For patients in hospital, therefore, who have been subject to many awakenings during the night, their subjective feelings of sleepiness the following day could be said to have some relevance in reflecting the quality of their sleep the night before.

There are reports that if subjects are deprived of REM sleep, that in their recovery sleep after the deprivation they have excessive amounts of REM sleep to make up for what they have lost. This is called REM rebound. Such reports were particularly prominent in the 1970s, when patients' delirium in Intensive Care Units following open-heart surgery led researchers to believe that their REM sleep deprivation in the Intensive Care Unit was the reason this happened (Johns et al 1974, Orr and Stahl 1977). The features of REM rebound are said to include lurid dreams and physiological disturbances such as surges in blood pressure, rises in heart rate and irregularities of respiration all of which occur in REM sleep normally, but which are exaggerated in REM rebound (Parkes 1985). Medical studies of patients to see if REM rebound occurred did not find any proof of it (Johns et al 1974, Orr and Stahl 1977) but they concluded that the sleep of the patients they observed in the intensive care areas was so disturbed that REM sleep was suppressed and so was REM rebound (Orr and Stahl 1977). More recently, general sleep researchers have failed to show that REM rebound always occurs (Borbély 1986, page 166) and conclude that it is probably something which happens in some people and not in others.

Sleep Disorders

For years people who fall asleep in the day at inappropriate times have been the butt of jokes and caricature, the most famous being Charles Dickens' Joe, the fat boy in the *Pickwick Papers* who kept falling asleep. This phenomenon became known as the Pickwickian Syndrome. In recent years, sleep research has uncovered the existence of fairly common sleep disorders that account for the Pickwickian Syndrome, with the result that many sleep disorder centres have been founded in the USA and Europe. Horne (1988a) mourned the fact that as yet there are no such centres in Britain. These disorders result in disturbed sleep and daytime sleepiness. The most common among them are described below.

Obstructive Sleep Apnoea

Obstructive sleep apnoea is common in people who for some reason have a narrowing of the upper respiratory tract which involves a greater effort on inspiration. This induces the tissues and musculature, relaxed in sleep, to collapse, obstructing the airway. This condition is associated with stenosis of the nasal passages, a short mandible, or conditions which cause airway narrowing due to submucosal infiltration of the tongue and throat, such as obesity, acromegaly and hypothyroidism. The symptoms are loud snoring, followed by apnoea for anything up to a minute or more. The patient during this time will try to breathe without success, and then finally clear the airway with a loud snort and continue snoring until the next apnoeic episode (Douglas 1984, Kavey and Anderson 1986). This continues through the night, and, not surprisingly, disrupts the sleep cycle. The patient will feel sleepy during the day and keep having the urge to 'nod off'.

Central Sleep Apnoea

Central sleep apnoea results from a lack of contraction of the diaphragm and intercostal muscles, and/or a lack of respiratory drive. It is therefore associated with such conditions as neuromuscular disorders, thoraco-skeletal abnormalities, respiratory disease and brainstem disorders. It often occurs in conjunction with obstructive sleep apnoea, and is then called 'mixed apnoea' (Gross 1986, Douglas 1984). Both types of apnoea occur during the periodic breathing at sleep onset and during irregular breathing in REM sleep. There are frequent arousals in the sleep cycle induced by repetitive hypoxic and hypercapnic episodes. These episodes eventually cause a blunting of the chemo-receptors and the respiratory drive, secondary to the initial disorder (Douglas 1984).

Treatment of Obstructive and Central Sleep Apnoea

The treatment for these disorders is to treat the cause. Diagnosis can be helped by observant and knowledgeable nursing at night. The obstructive apnoeas can be treated with weight loss for obesity, and helping the patient to develop ways of not lying on his back. The patient should avoid alcohol and drugs that depress the respiratory drive, as this is associated with an increased frequency and duration of apnoeic episodes (Douglas 1984). Sometimes oxygen therapy is used but the reason why it reduces the number of apnoeic episodes is not clear (Douglas 1984). Continuous positive airway pressure (CPAP) administered nasally through a special mask, is very effective as a treatment (Hanning 1986, Douglas 1984), but sometimes tracheostomy is required (Gross 1986, Kavey 1986). Respiratory stimulants can be used in both the central and the obstructive apnoeas.

Narcolepsy Syndrome

Narcolepsy syndrome is a mixture of strange phenomena, the most obvious of which is the overwhelming need for sleep, even in the middle of the day. It is thought to be a disorder associated with REM sleep regulation. Sometimes it is accompanied by cataplexy, a form of sleep paralysis which involves a few seconds or minutes when the patient is unable to move, usually at the end of a period of sleep, i.e. in REM sleep. This may be associated with hypnogogic hallucinations, which are frightening visual/dream sequences. Narcolepsy syndrome and its phenomena may be hereditary, but can result from severe head injury or brain tumour (Gross 1986). The attacks are precipitated by sudden emotional events, including laughter, anger or startle. The patient may become socially withdrawn in an attempt to avoid attacks (Gross 1986).

Perceptive nursing can help initiate diagnosis of narcolepsy (and any more sinister underlying cause), which is confirmed by the occurrence of REM sleep in at least two daytime naps, and various sleep latency tests. Treatment is for the patient to have prophylactic naps during the day, and sometimes to take central nervous system stimulants. The attacks of sleep paralysis and hypnogogic hallucinations, which can be so frightening, can be terminated by a sudden noise or touching the patient (Gross 1986).

Insomnia

Insomnia is one of the most well-known of the sleep disorders. It is divided into the three categories of the sleep process:

1. Problems of sleep onset – when the person cannot fall asleep.
2. Problems of sleep maintenance – when there are frequent periods of wakefulness through the night.
3. Problems of early awakening – when the sleeper awakes at 4.00am–4.30am and cannot get back to sleep again.

The main causes of insomnia are often temporary, such as worry over a particular problem. However, it is associated with depressive illness. In this case patients awaken early and there are night wakings. EEG would show SWS depression (Kellerman 1981). Sometimes the cause of insomnia remains unexplained.

Illness and Sleep

Since ancient classical times sleep has been associated with notions of healing, but its interaction with particular disease states has only more recently been researched. With the advent of more sophisticated electronic monitoring devices and computerised techniques (Meanock et al 1983, Astrom et al 1989) research into sleep and various pathologies increasingly demonstrates that different illnesses disrupt sleep in their own characteristic ways, and that conversely sleep can interact with disease states to exacerbate or ameliorate symptoms.

Pain

Pain as an unpleasant stimulus is an important cause of disturbed sleep. Sleep deprivation or disturbance can enhance pain. It has been shown that there is a particular syndrome, the 'fibrositis syndrome', associated with a specific EEG alpha rhythm arousal disorder within stages 2, 3 and 4 NREM sleep (Moldofsky et al 1984). Those afflicted describe their sleep as light and/or restless, and they awaken feeling unrefreshed with pains, stiffness, lethargy and physical exhaustion. Often they have been involved in some stressful or frightening event prior to the onset of their symptoms. When sleep was disturbed in normal subjects in a laboratory, they exhibited similar symptoms, as well as the EEG disturbance (Moldofsky and Scarisbrick 1976), and these findings have been repeated in people who are subject to sleep disturbance by environmental noise (Tarnopolsky et al 1980).

Arthritis

Moldofsky (1986b) suggests that the 'fibrositis syndrome' is the aetiology for the morning generalised pain and stiffness in patients in acute episodes of arthritis who have their sleep disrupted by joint pains. In primary osteo-arthritis similar symptoms have been found if sleep is disturbed (Moldofsky et al 1987). Leigh et al (1988) showed that osteoarthritic patients had more stage 1 sleep than controls and suggested that if sleep disturbance is such it could be seen as the indication for arthroplasty or other surgical intervention.

Asthma

Many asthmatic patients have increased broncho-constriction at night, particularly between 4am and 6am, when the most REM sleep occurs. Circadian rhythms are thought to play a role, as they do in REM sleep, however, it is possible that REM sleep causes changes in airway vagal tone (Catterall et al 1986, Shapiro et al 1986). Many asthmatic patients therefore waken with the impression of dreaming with an asthma attack, but may have little recollection of the dream content, because of the events surrounding the asthma attack itself (Monday et al 1987). This sensation of vivid dreaming without any content has been named 'white dreaming', and it has been argued that it is a defence mechanism against the type of material in the dreams. Psychotherapy studies have found dreams of asthmatics to be closely related to death anxiety, involving content of the patient drowning or being strangled, or undergoing some other suffocating experience similar to an asthma attack (Monday et al 1987).

Snoring and asthma are not happy bed-fellows. Shu Chan et al (1988) in a study of the use of nasal continuous positive airway pressure (nCPAP) in patients with snoring and asthma found that all patients reported a marked improvement in their asthma symptoms on waking and during the following day. It was hypothesised that the upper airway obstruction that resulted in the snoring was also a chronic irritant to the underlying asthma. The nCPAP was thought to result in improvement because it stabilised the upper airway and removed the trigger for broncho-constriction. The implication for nursing asthmatic patients who snore at night is that this is an important factor in the patients' aetiology and should be prevented by positioning; as well as being reported to medical staff with a view to a new approach to treatment.

Epilepsy

Epileptic attacks can be induced by sleep deprivation and by sleep itself, through extremely complex pathways, which are not yet fully understood. Temporal lobe epilepsy seems to be the most common form induced by sleep, be the seizures grand mal or petit mal (Parkes 1985).

The interictal EEG phenomena of epilepsy are known to change with the various sleep stages (Kellaway 1985, Autret et al 1987), but as yet the precise predictive nature of the changes that occur are not known. In a survey of the self-reports of epileptic patients' sleep, those patients with the most frequent fits reported the most disturbed sleep in terms of sleep onset latency, numbers of times they woke in the night, their experiences of nightmares and sleep walking, and feeling less well rested in the morning (Hoeppner et al 1984).

Parkinson's Disease

In Parkinson's disease fragmented sleep is common. Parkinson's disease causes prolonged sleep onset latency, more awakenings and less total sleep time. With treatment this improves. The tremor disappears during sleep, and patients' symptoms are initially improved after a good night's sleep (Parks 1985). Sleep apnoea syndrome has been observed, and it has been queried that it is part of the aetiology of sudden death in the middle of the night among these patients (Hardie et al 1986). The symptoms of Parkinsonism as well as the sleep disturbance improve with dopaminergic therapy (Askenasy and Yahr 1985).

Neuromuscular Disorders

All neuromuscular disorders can result in hypopnoea and apnoea at night in particular during REM sleep. Whilst various forms of ventilatory support have been devised over the years, in particular negative pressure ventilation devices (such as the 'iron lung') which can be used in the home, it has been proven that nasal positive pressure ventilation (nCPAP) is now the treatment of choice in neuromuscular disorders. It stabilises the upper airway and rib cage, whereas in negative pressure ventilation the airway can collapse, particularly in REM sleep when muscle relaxation exacerbates the pre-existing neuro-muscle weakness (Ellis et al 1987).

Diabetes

The research into diabetes and sleep has concentrated mainly on patients with diabetic autonomic neuropathy, where the incidence of sudden death during the night is relatively common (Catterall et al 1984). This has led researchers to think that such deaths may be related to respiratory arrests during sleep. Catterall et al (1984) found no evidence to support this theory, but Mondini and Guilleminault (1985) selected diabetic patients very carefully from both type 1 (insulin-dependent) and type 2 (late-onset, non-insulin dependent) groups, and found that breathing irregularities in Stages 3 and 4 NREM sleep (where breathing is normally regular) were much more common in the lean type 1 diabetics especially if they also had neuropathy, and that heart-rate adaptation to the resultant hypoxia was blunted or absent. They therefore concluded that these factors may contribute to the sudden deaths during sleep of insulin-dependent patients with diabetic neuropathy.

Myxoedema

Patients with untreated hypothyroidism do not have the same amount of SWS as normal controls. This improves with treatment. REM sleep appears to be unaffected. Myxoedema is strongly associated with snoring and obstructive sleep apnoea (Gross 1986, Hanning 1986) because of the thickening of the tissues in the upper airway which occurs as part of the pathology. Mackay et al (1984) found in a polysomnographic study of newly diagnosed patients with myxoedema that five out of the total of nine patients had episodes of sleep apnoea and had grossly disturbed sleep EEGs. The episodes of apnoea were found to be predominantly central in type (showing no evidence of movement of the chest wall) as well as obstructive. When these same patients had been treated and were euthyroid, their sleep and breathing returned to normal. The researchers in this study suggested that the sleep apnoea in hypothyroid patients is due to central changes, as well as to those in the upper airway.

Cardiac Disease

Research for many years has shown that there is a correlation between REM sleep and pathological cardiac events such as angina, dysrhythmias and myocardial infarction (Knowlin 1965, King 1973). This was thought to be due to the surges in blood pressure that occur during REM sleep, and it has since been demonstrated that the autonomic surges that are associated with this stage of sleep seem to lead to extra oxygen demand and consequent myocardial ischaemia (Quyyumi et al 1984, Zemaityté et al 1984, 1986).

Patients after acute myocardial infarction have been shown to have more SWS on their sleep EEG than normal on nights 3–9, and also to sleep a lot more in the day-time (Broughton and Baron 1978). This was shown to occur on both the intensive care unit, where patients were first monitored, and when they went to the general ward. It was also found that angina in the post-infarction phase seemed to occur more frequently in SWS sleep as opposed to REM sleep on nights 4 and 5. The fact that patients after myocardial infarction seem to need so much sleep, which could have an innate physiological cause, indicates that their nursing management should enhance what Nature indicates is best.

Cardiac Disease and Back Pain

The sight of cardiac patients breathless and distressed in the middle of the night is one that is familiar to many nurses on acute medical wards. Usually the patient has been lying down and the pressure in the right atrium has risen sufficiently to cause heart failure and pulmonary oedema. In spinal stenosis it has been reported that patients who also have a tendency to right heart failure, can be woken in the night with lumbosacral pain (Laban 1984). This is because the increased right atrial pressure, exacerbated by the supine position, gets transmitted through the paravertebral plexus to create venous distension, stasis and hypoxia in the epidural plexus, and the area of the stenosis. Pain results which wakens the patient. This demonstrates the interplay of various disease entities which can present symptoms exacerbated by or disruptive of the patient's sleep.

Chronic Obstructive Pulmonary Disease

Patients with chronic bronchitis and emphysema are at particular risk during sleep because of the natural alteration in breathing that occurs, particularly in REM sleep. Patients with chronic obstructive pulmonary diseases commonly show periods of oxygen desaturation during sleep, which are most frequent during REM sleep (Cormick et al 1986, Fletcher et al 1987). It has been shown that this is due to paralysis of the accessory muscles of respiration, in particular the scalene and sternocleidomastoid muscles, which occurs during REM sleep. This leaves the overworked respiratory muscles of the chronic bronchitic patient to work inadequately on their own (Johnson and Remmers 1984). The effect of the hypoxic episodes is to raise pulmonary arterial pressure, and some authorities have suggested that this results in the development over time of cor-pulmonale (Douglas 1984).

Not all patients with chronic obstructive pulmonary disease suffer oxygen desaturation at night. Manni et al (1988) found that patients who had less severe disease did not lose their oxygenation in the same way because their sleep was so fragmented, with a lot of arousals and awakenings. This meant that they rarely had REM sleep. It was suggested that the apparently poor sleep of such patients was a protection against nocturnal hypoxia.

Doctors and nurses tend to restrict sleep medication and analgesia at night in patients with chronic chest disease for fear of reducing the respiratory drive still further. Symptoms such as dyspnoea, cough and troublesome secretions together with aggressive medical treatments, physiotherapy and nursing interventions often lead to sleep deprivation. However, evidence is emerging that sleep deprivation can adversely affect respiratory effort and significantly blunten the hypercapnic ventilatory response (Cooper et al 1982, White et al 1983). These events, occurring in patients with chronic respiratory disease, will therefore compound the existing pathology and lead to hypoventilation (Cooper et al 1982, White et al 1983). Nursing interventions in this situation should therefore enable the patient to sleep if possible, whilst close observation and supportive therapy is maintained.

Renal Disease

Whilst uraemia is recognised as a cause of drowsiness in renal failure, medical research has demonstrated that a proportion of these patients suffer from sleep apnoea syndrome. It has therefore been suggested that sleep apnoea syndrome be suspected in patients with chronic renal failure and excessive drowsiness (Kimmel et al 1989, Millman et al 1985). Some of the effects of renal failure, such as proteinuria in the nephrotic syndrome, have been reversed by treatment of the sleep apnoea syndrome (Chaudhary et al 1988); whilst in uraemic patients, dialysis has improved their sleep apnoea (Fein et al 1987).

Nursing research into patients' sleep in renal failure has been somewhat complicated by the numerous possible causes for the patients to feel fatigued which are related to their disease rather than to their sleep (Srivastava 1986). In a study to develop a sleep instrument for patients with end-stage renal disease (ESRD) (Needham Moore 1989), it was found that patients all acknowledged being woken by a wide variety of physical complaints associated with the illness, such as muscle twitching, restless legs, itching and dry skin. Half of the patients in the sample needed anti-inflammatory medication for 'aches and pains', and half the sample showed a 'mild to moderate' degree of depression. This was a very small sample conducted as a pilot study, but is one of very few nursing studies into particular disease states and sleep.

Gastro-intestinal Disorders

Hypersecretion of acid occurs at night in patients with duodenal ulcer (Lam 1984). This also occurs during stressful life events; therefore, in patients who have a tendency for this disorder, an admission to hospital could prove a potent trigger to symptoms which are manifest at night. The sleeping position of patients with reflux has long been recognised as best with the bed-head raised or supportive pillows and this position has also been shown to improve the effects of medication (Harvey et al 1987).

Conclusion

Sleep it would seem has the potential to aid healing and reduce distress. Whilst researchers continue to try to unlock the secrets surrounding the function of sleep, nurses cannot ignore the essential message of sleep research which is that people need their sleep. Disturbed sleep leading to sleep deprivation is common in hospital. The reasons for it differ according to the pathology, environment and individual factors.

If patients are to have the best possible sleep at night the first five hours would appear to be the most important for their restorative function, both in terms of the effects on the brain, and for the physiological events associated with SWS and REM sleep. This essential sleep has been described as 'core' sleep (Horne 1988a). The first 3–5 hours should therefore ideally be uninterrupted. If care is required to change wet beds or change position, it may well help enhance sleep quality. The fact that many patients will need longer than 5 hours of sleep for comfort, for their 'optional' sleep, should be something all ward routines should accommodate, for besides the comfort needs, illness may increase the amount of time patients need to sleep.

References

Adam K (1980) Sleep is a restorative process and a theory to explain why. *Progress in Brain Research*, **53**, 289–305.

Adam K and Oswald I (1977) Sleep is for tissue restoration. *Journal of the Royal College of Physicians*, **11**, 376–388.

Agnew H W, Webb W B and Williams R L (1967) Comparison of Stage 4 and REM sleep deprivation. *Perceptual Motor Skills*, **24**, 66–879.

Ambrosini M V, Sadile A G, Gironi Carnevale U A, Mattiaccio M and Guiditta A (1988) The sequential hypothesis in sleep function. 1. Evidence that the structure of sleep depends on the nature of the previous waking experience. *Physiology and Behaviour*, **43**, 325–3337.

Aserinsky E and Kleitman N (1953) Regular occurring periods of eye motility and concomitant phenomena during sleep. *Science*, **118**, 273–274.

Askenasy J J M and Yahr M D (1985) Reversal of sleep disturbance in Parkinson's disease by anti-Parkinsonian therapy: a preliminary study. *Neurology*, **35**, 527–532.

Astrom C and Jochumsen (1989) Decrease in delta sleep in growth hormone deficiency assessed by a new power spectrum analysis. *Sleep*, **12**, 6, 508–515.

Astrom C and Lindholm J (1990) Growth hormone deficient young adults have decreased deep sleep. *Neuroendocrinology*, **51**, 1, 82–84.

Autret A, Lucas B, Laffont F, Bertrand P, Degiovanni E and De Toffol B (1987) Two distinct classifications of adult epilepsies: by time of seizures, by sensitivity of the interictal paroxysmal activities to sleep and waking. *Electroencephalography and Clinical Neurophysiology*, **66**, 211–218.

Bixler E O and Vela-Bueno A (1987) Normal sleep: patterns and mechanisms. *Seminars in Neurology*, **7**, 3, 227–235.

Bonnet M H (1986a) Auditory thresholds during continuing sleep. *Biological Psychology*, **22**, 3–10.

Bonnet M H (1986b) Performance and sleepiness following moderate sleep disruption and Slow Wave Sleep deprivation. *Physiology and Behaviour*, **37**, 915–918.

Borbély A (1986) *Secrets of Sleep*. English translation. London: Penguin.

Broughton R and Baron R (1978) Sleep patterns in the intensive care unit and on the ward after myocardial infarction. *Electroencephalography and Clinical Neurophysiology*, **45**, 348–360.

Campbell S S (1984) Duration and placement of sleep in a 'disentrained' environment. *Psychophysiology*, **21**, 1, 106–113.

Carter D (1984) *Sleeping soundly? Sleep and the low-dependency hospital patient.* Unpublished MSc thesis. University of Glasgow.

Catterall J R, Calverley P M, Ewing D J, Shapiro C M, Clarke B F and Douglas N J (1984) Breathing, sleep and diabetic autonomic neuropathy. *Diabetes*, **33**, 1025–1027.

Catterall J R, Rhind G B, Stewart I C, Whyte K F, Shapiro C M and Douglas N J (1986) Effect of sleep deprivation on overnight bronchoconstriction in nocturnal asthma. *Thorax*, **41**, 676–680.

Chaudhary B A, Siklar A H, Chaudhary T K, Kolbeck R C and Speir W A Jr. (1988) Sleep apnoea, proteinuria and nephrotic syndrome. *Sleep*, **11**, 1, 69–74.

Closs S J (1988) *A nursing study of sleep on surgical wards.* Report for the Scottish Home and Health Dept. University of Edinburgh.

Cooper K R and Phillips B A (1982) Effect of short-term sleep loss on breathing. *Journal of Applied Physiology*, **53**, 855–858.

Cormick W, Olson L G, Hensley M J and Saunders N A (1986) Nocturnal hypoxaemia and quality of sleep in patients with chronic obstructive lung disease. *Thorax*, **41**, 846–854.

Dijk D J, Beersma D G M, Daan S and Lewy A J (1989) Bright morning light advances the human circadian system without affecting NREM sleep homeostasis. *American Journal of Physiology*, **256**, R106–R111.

Dodds E J (1980) *Slept well? A study of ward activity and nurse patient interaction at night.* Unpublished MSc thesis. University of Surrey.

Douglas N J (1984) Control of breathing during sleep. *Clinical Science*, **67**, 465–471.

Ellis B W, Johns M W, Lancaster R, Raptopoulos P, Angelopoulos N and Priest R G (1981) The St. Mary's Hospital Sleep Questionnaire: a study of reliability. *Sleep*, **4**, 93–97.

Ellis B W, Bye P T P, Bruderer J W and Sullivan C E (1987) Treatment of Respiratory Failure during Sleep in Patients with Neuromuscular Disease. *American Review of Respiratory Disease*, **135**, 148–152.

Empson J E (1989) *Sleep and Dreaming.* London: Faber and Faber.

Fass G (1971) Sleep, drugs and dreams. *American Journal of Nursing*, **71**, 12, 2316–2320.

Fein A M, Neiderman M S, Imbriano L and Rosen H (1987) Reversal of sleep apnoea in uraemia by dialysis. *Archives of International Medicine*, **147**, 7, 1355–1356.

Fletcher E C, Miller J, Divine G W, Fletcher J G and Miller T (1987) Nocturnal oxyhaemaglobin desaturation in COPD patients with arterial oxygen tensions above 60mm Hg. *Chest*, **92**, 4, 604–608.

Frankel B L, Coursey R D, Buchbinder R and Snyder F (1976) Recorded and reported sleep in chronic and primary insomnia. *Archives of General Psychiatry*, **33**, 615–623.

Gross P T (1986) Evaluation of sleep disorders. *Medical Clinics of North America*, **70**, 6, 1349–1360.

Hanning C D (1986) Sleep and breathing: 'to sleep perchance to breathe'. *Intensive Care Nursing*, **2**, 8–15.

Hardie R J, Efthimiou J and Stern G M (1986) Respiration and sleep in Parkinson's disease. (Letter). *Journal of Neurology Neurosurgery and Psychiatry*, **49**, 11, 1326.

Hartmann J (1973) *The Functions of Sleep.* London: Yale University Press.

Harvey R F, Hadley N, Gill T R, Beats B C, Gordon P C, Long D E, Macpherson R I and Tottle A J (1987) Effects of sleeping with the bedhead raised and of Ranitidine in patients with severe peptic oesophagitis. *The Lancet*, 21 November 1987, 1200–1203.

Hayter J (1983) Sleep behaviours in older persons. *Nursing Research*, **32**, 4, 242–246.

Hilton B A (!976) Quantity and quality of patients' sleep and sleep-disturbing factors in a respiratory intensive care unit. *Journal of Advanced Nursing*, **1**, 453–468.

Hoeppner J B, Garron D C and Cartwright R D (1984) Self-reported sleep disorder symptoms in epilepsy. *Epilepsia*, **25**, 4, 434–437.

Horne J A (1983) Human sleep and tissue restitution: some qualifications and doubts. *Clinical Science*, **65**, 569–578.

Horne J A (1988a) *Why we Sleep: The Functions of Sleep in Humans and other Mammals*. Oxford: Oxford University Press.

Horne J A (1988b) The substance of sleep. *New Scientist*. **1594**, 60–62.

Horne J A and Ostberg O (1976) A self-assessment questionnaire to determine morningness and eveningness in human circadian rhythms. *International Journal of Chronobiology*, **4**, 97–110.

Irwin H P (1989) *A comparative study of the self-reported sleep patterns of medical patients on Nightingale wards with and without partitions*. Unpublished MSc thesis. University of Manchester.

Jarrett D B, Miewald J M and Kupfer D J (1990) Recurrent depression is associated with a persistent reduction in sleep-related growth hormone secretion. *Archives of General Psychiatry*, **47**, 2, 113–118.

Johns M W (1977) Validity of subjective reports of sleep latency in normal subjects. *Ergonomics*, **20**, 6, 683–690.

Johns M W and Doré C (1978) Sleep at home and in the laboratory: disturbance by recording procedures. *Ergonomics*, **21**, 5, 325–330.

Johns M W, Large A A, Masterton J P and Dudley H A F (1974) Sleep and delirium after open heart surgery. *British Journal of Surgery*, **61**, 377–381.

Johnson J E (1986) Sleep and bed-time routines of non-institutionalised aged women. *Journal of Community Health Nursing*, **3**, 3, 117–125.

Johnson M W and Remmers J E (1984) Accessory muscle activity during sleep in chronic obstructive pulmonary disease. *Journal of Applied Physiology*, **57**, 4, 1011–1017.

Karacan, I, Thornby J I, Anch A M and Williams R L (1978) The effects of high ambient temperature on the sleep of young men. *Sleep Research*, **7**, 171.

Kavey N B and Altshuler K Z (1979) Sleep in herniorraphy patients. *American Journal of Surgery*, **138**, 682–687.

Kavey N B and Anderson A (1986) Why every patient needs a good night's sleep. *RN*, December 1986, 16–19.

Kellaway P (1985) Sleep and epilepsy. *Epilepsia*, **26** (Suppl. 1), S15–S30.

Kemp J (1984) Nursing at night. *Journal of Advanced Nursing*, **9**, 217–223.

Kimmel P L, Miller G and Mendelson W B (1989) Sleep apnoea syndrome in chronic renal disease. *American Journal of Medicine*, **86**, 3, 308–314.

King M J, Zir L M, Kaltman A J and Fox A C (1973) Variant angina associated with angiographically demonstrated coronary artery spasm and REM sleep. *American Journal of Medical Science*, **265**, 419–422.

Knowlin B J, Troyer W G, Collins W S, Silverman G, Nicholas C R, McIntosh H D, Estes E H and Bogdonoff M D (1965) The association of nocturnal angina with dreaming. *Annals of International Medicine*, **63**, 1040–1046.

Kreuger J M, Walter J, Dinarello C A, Wolff S M and Chedid L (1984) Sleep promoting effects of endogenous pyrogen (Interleukin–1). *American Journal of Physiology*, **246**, R994–R999.

Kreuger J M, Karaszewski J W, Davenne D and Shoham S (1986) Somnogenic muramyl peptides. *Federal Proceedings*, **45**, 11, 2552–2555.

Laban M M (1984) 'Vespers curse' Night pain – the bane of hypnos. *Archives of Physical Medicine and Rehabilitation*, **65**, 501–503.

Lam S K (1984) Pathogenesis and pathophysiology of duodenal ulcer. *Clinical Gastroenterology*, **13**, 2, 447–472.

Leigh T J, Hindmarch I, Bird H A and Wright B F (1988) Comparison of sleep in osteoarthritic patients and age and sex matched healthy controls. *Annals of the Rheumatic Diseases*, **47**, 40–42.

Mackay D, Cooper R A, Bradbury S, Gaukrodger D J, Proswe K and Van'T Hoff W (1984) Sleep apnoea in myxoedema. *Journal of the Royal College of Physicians*, **18**, 4, 248–252.

Manfredi R L and Kales A (1987) Clinical neuropharmacology of sleep disorders. *Seminars in Neurology*, **7**, 3, 286–295.

Manni R, Cerveri I, Bruschi C, Zoia C and Tartara A (1988) Sleep and oxyhaemaglobin desaturation patterns in chronic obstructive pulmonary diseases. *European Neurology*, **28**, 275–278.

Meanock C I, Guyatt A R and Cumming G (1983) The assessment of nocturnal oxygen saturation. *Clinical Science*, **65**, 507–513.

Meddis R M (1983) The evolution of sleep. In Mayes A (ed.) *Sleep Mechanisms and Functions in Humans and Animals: an Evolutionary Perspective*. London: Van Nostrand Reinhold.

Millman R P, Kimmel P L, Shore E T and Wasserstein A B (1985) Sleep apnoea in haemodialysis patients: the lack of testosterone effect on its pathogenesis. *Nephron*, **40**, 4, 407–410.

Moldofsky H and Scarisbrick P (1976) Induction of neuraesthenic musculo-skeletal pain syndrome by selective sleep stage deprivation. *Psychosomatic Medicine*, **38**, 35–44.

Moldofsky H, Tullis C, Lue F A, Quance G and Davidson J (1984) Sleep-related myoclonus in rheumatic pain modulation disorder (Fibrositis Syndrome) and in excessive daytime somnolence. *Psychosomatic Medicine*, **46**, 2, 145–151.

Moldofsky H, Lue F A, Eisen J, Keystone E and Gorczynski R M (1986a) The relationship of Interleukin–1 and immune functions to sleep in humans. *Psychosomatic Medicine*, **48**, 5, 309–318.

Moldofsky H (1986b) Sleep and musculo-skeletal pain. *American Journal of Medicine*, **81** (Suppl. 3A), 85–89.

Moldofsky H, Lue F A and Saskin P (1987) Sleep and morning pain in primary osteoarthritis. *Journal of Rheumatology*, **14**, 1, 124–128.

Monday J, Montplaisir J and Malo J L (1987) Dream process in asthmatic subjects with nocturnal attacks. *American Journal of Psychiatry*, **144**, 5, 638–640.

Mondini S and Guillemnault C (1985) Abnormal breathing patterns during sleep in diabetes. *Annals of Neurology*, **17**, 4, 391–395.

Moore-Ede M C (1983) The circadian timing system in mammals: two pacemakers preside over many secondary oscillators. *Federal Proceedings*, **42**, 2802–2808.

Morgan K (1987) *Sleep and Ageing*. London: Croom Helm.

National Health Service Management Consultancy Services (1987) *Study of the Night Nursing Services*. Report No. 2/87. London: DHSS.

Needham Moore M (1989) Development of a sleep-awake instrument for use in a chronic renal population. *ANNA Journal*, **16**, 1, 15–19.

Orr W C and Stahl M L (1977) Sleep disturbances after open heart surgery. *American Journal of Cardiology*, **39**, 196–201.

Oswald I (1980) *Sleep* (4th edn) London: Penguin.

Parkes J D (1985) *Sleep and its Disorders*. Philadelphia: W B Saunders.

Phillips G D and Cousins M J (1986) Neurological mechanisms of pain and the relationship of pain, anxiety and sleep. In Cousins M J and Phillips G D (eds) *Acute Pain Management. Clinics in Critical Care Medicine*, 21–48. Edinburgh: Churchill Livingstone.

Quyyumi A A, Wright C A, Mockus I J and Fox K M (1984) Mechanisms of nocturnal angina pectoris: importance of increased myocardial oxygen demand in patients with severe coronary artery disease. *The Lancet*, 2nd June, 1207–1209.

Shapiro C M, Catterall J R, Montgomery I, Raab G M and Douglas N J (1986) Do asthmatics suffer bronchoconstriction during rapid eye movement sleep? *British Medical Journal*, **292**, 3rd May, 1161–1164.

Shu Chan C, Woolcock A J and Sullivan C E (1988) Nocturnal asthma: the role of snoring and obstructive sleep apnoea. *American Review of Respiratory Diseases*, **137**, 1502–1504.

Smith C and Kelly G (1988) Paradoxical sleep deprivation applied two days after end of training retards learning. *Physiology and Behaviour*, **43**, 213–216.

Srivastava R H (1986) Fatigue in the renal patient. *ANNA Journal*, **13**, 5, 246–249.

Tarnopolsky A, Watkins A G and Hand D J (1980) Aircraft noise and mental health. 1. Prevalence of individual symptoms. *Psychological Medicine*, **10**, 683–698.

Webb W W (1982) Sleep in older persons: Sleep structures of 50–60-year-old men and women. *Journal of Gerontology*, **37**, 5, 581–586.

Webb W B (1983) Theories in modern sleep research. In Mayes A (ed.) *Sleep Mechanisms and Functions in Humans and Animals: an Evolutionary Perspective.* London: Van Nostrand Reinhold.

White D P, Douglas N J, Pickett A, Zwillich C W and Weil J V (1983) Sleep deprivation and the control of ventilation. *American Review of Respiratory Diseases*, **128**, 984–986.

Williams D H (1971) Sleep and disease. *American Journal of Nursing*, **71**, 12, 2321–2324.

Wright J and Koulack D (1987) Dreams and contemporary stress: a disruption-avoidance-adaptation model. *Sleep*, **10**, 2, 172–179.

Zemaityté D, Varoneckas G and Sokolov E (1984) Heart rhythm during sleep in ischaemic heart disease. *Psychophysiology*, **21**, 3, 290–298.

Zemaityté D, Varoneckas G, Plauska K and Kaukenas J (1986) Components of the heart rhythm power spectrum in wakefulness and individual sleep stages. *International Journal of Psychophysiology*, **4**, 129–141.

Zepelin H, Mcdonald C S and Zammit G K (1984) Effects of age on auditory awakening thresholds. *Journal of Gerontology*, **39**, 3, 294–300.

Chapter 4
Nursing Intervention at Night

Anne Cawthorn and Kevin Hope

People need sleep – without it we become irritable and anti-social, indeed our very ability to think coherently is impaired. Closs (1988) presents the evidence for its beneficial effects on healing, Torrance (1990) promotes the case of increased tissue repair occurring during sleep whilst Oswald (1984) argues that sleep contributes to both physical and psychological restoration. Further examples are presented elsewhere.

As a consequence, any factor which impedes the person's ability to sleep should be of concern to the nurse at night. Several authors have identified such factors. Willis (1989) focuses on environmental problems, like the telephone ringing, as well as nursing activities such as the recording of observations, pressure area care and drug administration which all have potentially negative effects on sleeping. Webster (1986) points to extraneous noise such as nurses talking, equipment being moved and the often unfamiliar distractions of others asleep. In addition, she highlights the fact that in hospital ambient temperatures are usually higher than those the patient is used to, which is in itself problematic. As well as these external factors, Webster draws attention to the intrinsic aspects of sleeplessness, namely discomfort, pain and anxiety.

Stead (1985) is critical of managerial issues particularly the work that night staff are required to do before the day-staff's arrival, a point Carter (1985) underlines when she identifies that one problem is the lack of time available for patients to sleep.

Beaumont (1988) offers '5 P's' as a framework for recognising factors which have a detrimental effect on sleep. These are:

1. Physical – those associated with disease, e.g. musculoskeletal problems or dyspnoea.
2. Physiological – e.g. jet lag, shift working and those related to one's sleeping environment such as temperature, humidity and noise.
3. Psychological – e.g. loneliness, frustration, worry, insecurity, separation and fear.

4. Psychiatric – those related to mental health problems.
5. Pharmacological – e.g. the negative effects of drugs such as beta blockers as well as nicotine, caffeine and alcohol all of which have been associated with insomnia.

There is, then, a wealth of literature which identifies in quite specific terms the problems that patients can experience when trying to sleep. What is it that nurses can do to alleviate such problems? A reasonable starting point might be to identify what it is we mean by a nursing intervention.

Traditionally, nursing has followed a path directed by the medical model of care which, as Pearson (1988) argues, leads to the routinisation of nursing care delivery. In parallel, technical tasks tend to be viewed more positively and those nurses involved in such tasks achieve higher status within the profession.

More recently, however, there has been a definite movement towards the concept of nursing as therapeutic in its own right. Ersser (1988), for example, states that therapeutic nursing can be described as:

'those approaches used by nurses which have an overriding tendency to produce subjective feelings of improvement in the person being helped, whether or not a demonstrable change is evident.'

Wright (1990) argues that nursing is about offering concerned, compassionate and creative caring pointing out that 'basic' nursing does not exist. Instead, he maintains that what we have historically delegated to the realms of simple tasks are in fact 'highly complex, intricate and valuable in their own right'. Pearson (1988) argues that the status of the skilled nurse at the patient's side needs to be seen as equal to that of the nurse involved in hi-tech care, e.g. ensuring clean sheets to promote comfort should have the same professional equivalence as understanding how to use an intravenous pump.

In trying to identify and promote excellence in the delivery of nursing care at night, we unashamedly take the view that nursing practice must encapsulate its artistic side if it is to be truly effective and consequently therapeutic. By this we mean those aspects of nursing care that are not particularly measureable. Instead, it is those parts of our role which are intricately interwoven with the notion of caring, about promoting the feelings of comfort and safety and with assisting people to put their trust in us. This does not happen just by chance.

It involves the skilful use of one's self in interpersonal relationships; it involves concentrating on the so-called basics of nursing and raising their importance in our own consciousness so that we begin to realise that such basics are in fact fundamental.

Nurses working at night should be able to identify with such a viewpoint. For too long their skills have been undervalued both within society and the profession for reasons the aforementioned authors identify. In countering this myth, we aim to underline how nurses can be therapeutic in the delivery of care by taking account of fundamental aspects of care, particularly at night when the potential for such intervention is arguably greater.

We have considered aspects of nursing care delivery as it pertains primarily to the provision of a therapeutic environment. This encapsulates elements of both ward and patient management.

Questioning Routines

Many patients can suffer from sleep disturbances due to the way they are managed during the night. In order to remedy this situation, nurses need to ask themselves three questions. What are they doing? Why are they doing it and who will benefit? If the answer to the last question is (at least in part) not the patient then this is the starting point for change to occur.

Walsh and Ford (1989) examine many nursing procedures and question whether much of what happens to patients is determined by what is convenient to nursing staff rather than what the patient wants. All too often nurses say that they have not got time but is too much time being spent on care which is ritualised and often unnecessary?

For example, decisions can be made about which observations and procedures can be performed during the day and which can be omitted at night. Such decisions can significantly influence whether or not the patient has a good night's sleep.

McMahon (1990) cites non-urgent intravenous blood transfusions as an example of a procedure which can sometimes be better planned. Ideally, if these were commenced in the morning and completed by the evening, this would eliminate patients being disturbed when recording observations.

Another example is the way work is organised throughout the night. We can perhaps all identify with the dawn scramble described by Walsh and Ford (1989) where everything is done before the day staff arrive. Indeed, one can recall patients being woken earlier because of the amount of work to be done! Who is this trying to please? Surely not the patient!

The 6am drug round could similarly be criticised as routine and ritualised. For some patients, stable blood levels are needed to ensure maximum effectiveness, therefore it is essential that their medication is received at fixed times (Walsh and Ford 1989). However, this is not the case for the majority of patients and their drug regime could commence later. Some wards have changed this practice with beneficial results and there is a case for others to follow suit.

Routines such as washing patients and early morning tea can all be done within a framework of individualised care. Many of those who wish to sleep can and should be left to do so, leaving the nurse time to attend to others.

Fortunately, nurses are beginning to question whether such practices are necessary, indeed justifiable in terms of individualised care. Many aspects can be changed by simply examining why we do it and again by organising the care over twenty-four hours. One obvious implication is that relationships between day and night staff need to be such that open discussion and questioning of practice is the norm so that changes in twenty-four hour care are facilitated. Internal rotation and the effects of clinical grading with its notion of 'twenty-four hour responsibility' have led to a more integrated approach to ward management in many areas. One happy consequence is the increased involvement of night staff in decision making.

Patients' Pre-Sleep Routine

Allowing patients to undertake their normal sleep routines may have a significant effect on how quickly they settle down to sleep. McMahon (1990) suggests that nurses need to assess patients' routines in order to establish individualised care that will give a 'normal' feel to the activity of going to bed.

Assessment needs to identify what helps as well as what hinders sleep. For example, if someone normally reads or watches television before going to sleep, then facilitating this activity may be helpful.

Another important factor is to maintain the person's previous dietary habits. Fordham (1986) points out that diet affects sleep, whilst Adam (1980) in her study concluded that a departure from a person's usual pattern of food intake in the evening impairs subsequent sleep.

For example, patients who are gaining weight tend to sleep longer and at a deeper level, whereas anorexic individuals or those losing weight sleep for shorter periods and have disrupted sleep. Each nurse will meet many patients who fit into this latter group for a variety of reasons. For example, very ill patients may not be receiving adequate daily calorific requirements to meet their body's demands as can be the case with cancer cachexia. Additionally, patients on a weight reducing diet and surgical patients who have had unnecessarily long periods of starving prior to surgery may also fit into this category.

Some patients are genuinely hungry later at night due to the final meal of the day being at around 6pm. As most wards now do not have facilities to provide snacks, patients who normally eat at bedtime will need to be encouraged to provide their own food. Storage of such food can be problematic particularly in the light of legislation applying to ward areas. This raises an interesting dilemma of how nurses gain access to food at times convenient to patients. This is especially relevant for those patients who are unable to depend on relatives supplying bedtime snacks.

Alongside meals, bedtime drinks are the subject of much debate in terms of their efficacy in promoting sleep. The timing of their provision can be dictated by nursing needs, i.e. when staff are available or when other care takes priority, and therefore may be given at inappropriate times. One solution might be the provision of drink-making facilities, which would allow suitable patients to make their own drinks as and when they need them. This also can give nurses time to attend to other patients requiring greater assistance. In doing so, they can then provide drinks to such patients on a more individualised basis pertinent to their needs.

Another important factor which tends to be underestimated is the effects of different types of drinks. Drinks such as tea, coffee and cola contain caffeine which is a stimulant and is therefore best avoided by people who have difficulty sleeping. However, as McMahon (1990) points out, if patients are used to having a regular supply of caffeine then to stop it will initiate withdrawal effects (e.g. headaches and disturbed sleep patterns) at least in the short term. Similarly, alcohol may help individuals to go to sleep quicker (i.e. shorten sleep latency) but can lead to early wakening and a feeling that the quality of sleep has been reduced.

Recent research by Morgan et al (1989) found that elderly insomniacs who drank tea at night on waking exacerbated their problem in two ways. Firstly, because the tea acted as a stimulant and secondly, disturbed again later on in order to pass urine. In the light of this information, nurses need to consider which drink is best given to a patient who wakes in the night so as not to reinforce this vicious cycle.

Beaumont (1988) suggests that milky drinks could aid sleep but research into its benefits are inconclusive. What is evident though is that such drinks do not appear to have any detrimental effect on sleep. Fordham (1986) suggests that what is beneficial is to maintain the patient's normal drink routine.

In conclusion, it would appear that if one alters the patient's pre-sleep dietary routine, this can lead to problems which may not otherwise have arisen. Therefore, time spent in providing individualised care prior to patients going to sleep may well reduce the need for nursing intervention later during the night.

Ward Environment

Another way that nurses can help to ensure that patients sleep is by managing the ward environment. The aim is simply to promote a therapeutic environment which not only helps the patient go to sleep but also helps them to remain alseep.

Noise

One important aspect which influences the environment is noise which is recognised as a major problem for patients who are trying to sleep. Ogilvie (1980) measured noise levels at night and found them to be those recommended for living rooms, not bedrooms. Certain noises are unavoidable such as that originating from traffic or emergency admissions, however, as McMahon (1990) suggests, much can be done to eradicate other disturbances. He puts them into three categories; noisy nurses, noisy equipment and noisy patients.

Nurses may be unaware of the amount of noise they make and therefore need to make a conscious effort to minimise the amount of noise created. Noise seems to carry more at night and nurses can linger in the false belief that their conversation is not disturbing anybody, particularly if it takes place at a nursing station for example or any area removed from the patients. Speaking in hushed tones is helpful.

Talking to patients at night is, of course, essential but problems may present when communicating with patients who have hearing difficulties particularly when one is trying to avoid disturbing other clients. McMahon (1990) suggests that cupping one's hands around the patient's ear when speaking can reduce disturbance for other patients. Another source of noise is nurses' shoes and Stead (1985) suggests that all night nurses should wear rubber soled shoes.

Equipment can create unwanted noise. Squeaky wheels on trolleys or commodes need attending to. Stead (1985) recommends that bedpan machines are not used at night whilst Kearns (1989) points out that simply taking time to explain to patients about what noise to expect at night is helpful. It would appear that realistic expectations of such disturbances can reduce the degree of discomfort perceived by patients. Fordham (1986) argues that night staff should not be alone in shouldering responsibility for reducing noise even though it occurs at night. Sometimes the solution is only available during the day, especially with regards to repair and maintenance of equipment. However, it is the night nurse's responsibility for initiating this process.

Noisy patients keep others awake. Every ward has a group of patients who snore, cough or call out. McMahon (1990) suggests that they could be grouped together in one area of the ward (although it is important to investigate why patients are being noisy). Obviously the ward layout will determine whether or not this is feasible. Similarly, paying attention to the positioning of patients can minimise the disturbance created by the arrival of somebody newly admitted.

One area worthy of particular attention is that associated with the management of the confused person, not least due to the degree of disturbance this can create. There is an increasing amount of literature on the subject, but little pertains to intervention at night when perhaps its incidence is, if not more frequent (and the clinical picture would indicate this to be the case), then certainly more disruptive.

Confused behaviour is a symptom, not an illness. It can be associated with a number of primary causes, e.g. dementia, depression, infection, malnutrition, dehydration, drugs and pain and can display itself in a number of ways, e.g.:

- poor memory
- disorientation in time, place or person
- reduced cognitive abilities
- impaired speech
- altered consciousness (drowsy, sleepless, over-alert)
- lability of mood
- restlessness, wandering
- disturbed sleep, e.g. reversed sleep pattern
- illusions, delusions and hallucinations.

It is important to realise though that health professionals and environmental factors can both create and exacerbate confused states. But what can nurses do at night?

Beneficial practice is characterised by taking time, listening and explaining carefully, physical contact and raised self-awareness. The reader is urged to explore therapies aimed specifically at the individual with dementia which provide information on strategies which the nurse at night may wish to consider. These are Reality Orientation (RO), Validation Therapy and Resolution Therapy.

There is common ground in such strategies for nurses to utilise, despite the different foci, and that is in responding to the feelings being expressed by the confused individual. If responses are sensitive and accompanied by positive regard for the individual's predicament, amelioration of confused behaviour can result.

What can happen though is that nurses look for the 'quick fix'. Sadly, all too often the answer chosen is to administer medication which tends to be a neuroleptic, that is drugs which are aimed at ameliorating psychotic symptoms as opposed to sedating individuals. In addition, the many varied and potentially drastic side effects are well documented, particularly in the elderly (Gomez and Gomez 1990).

The effects of the confused behaviour at night should not be understated, and this aspect of care can be improved. For example, how many times is it seen as appropriate to objectively record factors related to the confused episode? Stokes (1986) suggests an ABC assessment tool when attempting to deal with wandering or screaming and shouting as examples:

A – the activating event – when and where did the behaviour commence?
   Were there any preceding activities? What else was going on?
B – what behaviour occurred? Its form, length, content etc.
C – consequences? What action was taken? What was its effect?

Such an analysis can be very beneficial as such data gathering exercises frequently lead to the identification of appropriate strategies for intervention.

Physical and Psychological Safety

Another element of a therapeutic environment is that the patient will feel safe both physically and psychologically.

For example, it is easy to underestimate the skills required when trying to settle a patient down for the night whilst maintaining such feelings of safety. The amount of time required will vary from patient to patient, but if someone is rushed, their anxiety levels will be raised, resulting in negative effects on their ability to sleep. Consequently, times invested in settling somebody down will pay dividends.

But what does this mean? Ensuring comfort is important. Simple measures such as a soft pillow, a confortable mattress and the right amount of bed clothes are essential. A good ward manager will ensure that all of these are available for the night staff's use. In addition, allowing the patient to bring in their own pillows or soft sheets can be very beneficial. Psychological safety on the other hand can be promoted. An example of this is the provision of a nurse call system which will assist patients to feel secure, knowing that help will be readily available if required.

The promotion of relaxation and comfort through such measures as puffing up pillows may seem mundane and obvious, and Webster (1986) argues that such activities are often left to the unqualified nurse to instigate. Does this imply that such activities require less skill? Does not the simple act of positioning someone require a knowledge of the effects of illness so that a comfortable position is indeed achieved. For example, poor positioning of pillows around the face of a paralysed patient could not only be physically uncomfortable but indeed psychologically distressing.

As described earlier, 'basic' care is an anomaly – all care, if given professionally, will aim at alleviating distress.

Stress

Psychological safety can further be promoted by minimising patients' stress levels.

Stress can be viewed as resulting from the interplay of three areas. The environment, the interpretation of the environment and the behavioural response of the individual. At the individual level, stress can be reduced or eliminated by changing one's interpretation of the environment or the behavioural response associated with it (Deberry et al 1989). The nurse can be a very effective facilitator at this level.

For example, anxiety levels are raised by fear of the unknown. The hospital environment is very much a source of unknowns for many patients and as a consequence their perception of the environment can be, and often is, a stressful one. Behaviours, actions and equipment that nurses have become familiar with over time, as well as the use of shorthand phrases, have the potential to increase anxiety in the unknowing patient.

Imagine the patient experiencing for the first time a scene where a number of people are having infusions. Add to this the influence of dimmed lights so that the image is an unclear one and possibly distorted, then it is not too hard to imagine how this can appear frightening. This would appear particularly so to someone about to undergo surgery or who was admitted at night and not had the opportunity to be orientated to their surroundings.

Other occurrences can take on a more worrying perspective at night particularly as the combination of time to ponder and the influence of an unfamiliar environment can raise one's fears. For example, the death of a patient heightens awareness of our own mortality and the uncomfortable thoughts associated with such an event seem to penetrate consciousness more at quiet times. This can be made worse if patients have not had the opportunity to discuss their feelings openly.

An example of this would be the unsuccessful rescuscitation of a fellow patient. Most patients find this particularly stressful, and a nurse who allows patients to express their fears will be acting therapeutically. However, such an action can only take place if the patient is 'given permission' to voice their feelings.

Through such activity the nurse helps the patient to make sense of their environment for themselves. In addition she becomes aware of any need for information which, when met, should help to reduce anxiety.

Simply taking time to explain, in terms that are understandable, is a very effective method of helping the patient make sense of their environment.

However, it may be simple to do but one might question how effectively it is done. Cook (1991) criticises the use of jargon and abbreviations that nurses use when communicating with patients. Nurses' interpersonal skills vary and there is perhaps a case for measuring one's effectiveness. One way of doing this is to ask the patient to feedback their understanding of the situation.

Relaxation

The need to reduce anxiety levels, to promote comfort and the feeling of safety are paramount. Fortunately, there are avenues that the nurse might usefully explore which focus specifically on helping individuals to relax and minimise anxiety. This will consequently influence the behavioural response to stress.

Relaxation has been defined as 'a positively perceived state or response in which a person feels relief of tension or strain' (Sweeney 1978). It can be achieved by a variety of means, not all of which suit everybody. To be effective, therefore, the patient needs to feel comfortable with the technique utilised.

Methods include meditation, progressive muscular relaxation, applied relaxation training, autogenesis, hypnosis and imagery. Deberry et al (1989) maintain that such meditation–relaxation techniques evoke the opposite of the stress response and reduce sympathetic nervous system activity.

It is important to realise that relaxation training is a skill which by definition needs to be practised and can be improved upon.

Progressive muscular relaxation techniques are designed to help people to reduce muscular tension and become more sensitive towards tension in their body. Characteristically this is achieved by producing increased tension in a muscle group followed by relaxation. Obviously, therefore, there will be contra-indications, e.g. somebody with an abdominal wound will not benefit from increased muscular tension around the wound site. However, this should not detract from the potential benefits of such exercises focused on other parts of the body.

Nurses could act as facilitators for such activity, taking on the role of a leader or patients could undertake them as a self-help activity. Options are either that the patient could practise relaxation which they had learnt during the day or alternatively listen to relaxation exercises using headphones. Gournay (1988) suggests that between four and eight sessions from a therapist during the day would facilitate abbreviated sessions to be done at bedtime utilising tapes. Such options are less demanding of nurses' time but will require the necessary resources to be available. In addition, it is more likely that these skills would then be retained and could be used by the patient in the future to relieve anxiety.

Imagery is a method which can enhance relaxation. The aim is to provide the patient with an image which is pleasant and relaxing or provides an alternative to their current reality. It has many clinical applications and can be directed specifically at a problem area such as pain management. Its use in this context though is limited as to how it might promote relaxation. Terms used synonymously are imagination, visualisation and fantasy.

The nurse can facilitate 'passage' into a more pleasant mental environment either using their own description or the patient's imagination. Zahourek (1988) suggests using images the patient is already familiar with and that have positive connotations, e.g. a favourite beach. In addition, words which develop sensory responses to the images are helpful such as 'soft', 'peace' and 'comfort'. The following example highlights this.

'An anxious burned patient experiencing pain and unable to sleep went, mentally, to a lush green meadow. The sky was blue with puffy clouds that made interesting shapes. The mountain air was fresh and crisp, the birds were singing and in the distance a brook babbled. She rested on grass that felt like green velvet puff pillows, and watched the clouds drift by. Warm and secure, her cares were left behind. Relieved and less tense, she slept'. (Zahourek 1988)

The choice of patient for such an activity needs to be a sensitive one. Zahourek (1988) suggests that someone with imagination who is willing to listen and expects positive outcomes from the exercise is preferable being more effective with such a patient. As with progressive muscular relaxation, this exercise can be learnt during the day and repeated at night or alternatively, tapes can be used.

Holistic Health Practices

Another way of providing comfort is through the use of holistic health practices which view the patient as a whole looking at their physical, psychological, social and spiritual needs. Husband (1988) points out that 'excellence in nursing will only come about when we reject the dichotomy of mind and body and embrace holism and holistic healing'.

One way of doing this is by introducing complementary therapies into nursing practice. Rankin-Box (1988) promotes the term complementary (as opposed to alternative) which is defined as 'two or more things mutually complementing each other's deficiencies'. This fits into the philosophy of such practices which are not aimed at replacing conventional treatments but rather at complementing them.

Many nurses are beginning to discover how these therapies can enhance current nursing and medical practice. Whilst recognising that only some of these can be practised at night, many, if undertaken during the day, will have benefits which are sustained during the night, thereby promoting sleep.

All of these therapies require that the nurse be trained in their use, however, the opportunities to undertake such training are increasing.

Aromatherapy

Aromatherapy is perhaps the most popular form of complementary therapy and evidence of it successfully working has been demonstrated by Passant (1990) with the elderly, and Turton (1989) in the community. However, research into its uses seems to be scarce and nurses need to add to that which has been undertaken by Valnet (1980) and Tisserant (1988).

Wise (1989) describes aromatherapy as the controlled use of essential oils to produce health and relaxation. It works through a combination of the healing properties of the oils, their smell and the effects of touch. The oils can be used separately or together with massage. Tisserand (1988) describes aromatherapy without massage being like 'an orchestra without a conductor', however, having found the oils to have direct benefit on patient care their uses both alone and in conjunction with massage will be discussed.

The essential oils have different properties. Some are relaxing, others uplifting. Lavender, Sandalwood and Ylang-ylang have relaxing properties and these may prove useful in helping to promote sleep. Peppermint oil is useful for nauseated patients and Basil and Eucalyptus for patients with respiratory disorders. The oils can be added to patients' baths, inhaled in a bown of warm water or simply put on to a handkerchief or pillow case. Oils can also be used in a burner or an ioniser, but as the choice of essential oils is a personal taste and there are potential side effects, generalised use is not recommended.

Massage

Massage is well recognised as being beneficial to patients. Both Sims (1986) and Jackson (1987) have demonstrated that massaging without oils reduced anxiety and pain and helps patients to sleep. The same effects have also been demonstrated using aromatherapy massage (Cawthorn 1991).

The therapeutic benefits of touch should not be underestimated. Tisserand (1988) reminds us that conventional medicine has lost much of its close contact with patients and in some ways is becoming increasingly technological and dehumanised. We have left behind skills which, before the increases in technology, nurses turned to more readily when patients were stressed.

Touch can reassure the patient that they are accepted, that they are safe and are loved. Our need to be loved and touched is greater when we are stressed and ill (Tisserand 1988). This is particularly so with elderly or bereaved patients who are often deprived of touch.

An aromatherapy massage need not take long. A ten minute hand or foot massage can be very effective. In our experience, massage undertaken during the day is still effective at night. The properties of the oils are long lasting and, in addition, once the muscles have been relaxed patients seem to benefit that night.

Reflexology

Another therapy is reflexology which has been developed from ancient Chinese healing methods. It works using the principle that all major organs of the body can be treated by massaging specific energy points on the feet (Norman 1988). This is done by applying controlled pressure with the thumbs. Goodwin (1988) maintains that it works by inducing a state of relaxation which releases muscular and emotional tension, improving circulation and blood supply to vital organs. This in turn eliminates toxins and waste matter. Thomas (1989) has reported benefits with elderly patients specifically in contributing to the reduction of anxiety levels.

Pet Therapy

Pet therapy is an example of a therapy which if undertaken during the day can enhance sleep at night. It is becoming much more common as wards are either allowing pets to visit or are having cats or dogs as part of the ward environment, particularly on long stay wards. Patients benefit from the stroking and the therapeutic effects are those associated with touch.

Whilst recognising that there are other complementary therapies which are currently being introduced into practice, we accept that the field is too large to be covered adequately in this format. The reader is encouraged to pursue their enquiries in more comprehensive texts.

On the whole complementary therapies are safe if practised by nurses qualified in their use. It needs to be noted that all have possible side effects and that there are contra-indications for their use. Nurses need to be aware of these. However, the potential benefits far outweigh such aspects and their use in gaining recognition. They appear to enhance patient care and improve the perceived quality of such care.

In terms of their relevance to night staff, McMahon (1990) suggests that complementary therapies aid sleep by working at a number of different levels. Some have a hypnotic effect, others are relaxing and thereby put the patient in a better position to fall asleep, whilst the benefit of many may simply be as a result of time spent with patients.

Additionally, if this time results in counselling, it may resolve psychological discomforts. In a recent research study it was found that five out of twenty patients who were massaged entered into a formal counselling session (Cawthorn 1991). The closeness of the situation may help facilitate patients talking about their worries. (One implication is that nurses using complementary therapies may also need to feel confident in their counselling skills.)

It is unclear, in scientific terms, how such therapies are beneficial but as Tisserand (1988) asks, does this really matter? What perhaps matters more is that such practices convey an unquestioning acceptance to the patient by saying I am here, I have time and I care. If as a consequence, the patient feels better, this can only be for the good.

Conclusion

Wright (1990) maintains that the heart of nursing lies in caring, but this term is so very difficult to pin down. It has many components and in nursing terms goes beyond mere concern. Instead, he argues, 'nursing as a skilful, knowledgeable and caring concern for the well-being of another transcends mere helping to become healing'. In as much, nursing is therapeutic in its own right.

There are many areas were the nurse can seek to improve patient care if she adopts a therapeutic approach. Ersser (1988) for example, identifies five such areas.

We have promoted the view of nursing as therapeutic in its own right. In addition, we have examined several aspects of the night nurse's role and aimed to highlight ways in which the therapeutic element of each may be improved upon.

Whilst in no way is this an exhaustive or fully comprehensive analysis of nursing intervention at night, we hope that it might spur the reader on to review their practice and as a result make a change for the better.

References

Adam K (1980) Dietary habits and sleep after bedtime drinks. *Sleep*, **3**, 1, 47–58.

Beaumont G (1988) Sleep disorder-assessing five Ps cuts the needs for benzodiazepines. *Geriatric Medicine*, **18**, 3, 11–14.

Carter D (1985) In need of a good night's sleep. *Nursing Times*, **81**, 86, 24–26.

Cawthorn A (1991) *Effectiveness of Aromatherapy*. Unpublished research report.

Closs J (1988) Patients' sleep-wake rhythms in hospital. *Nursing Times*, **84**, 1, 48–50.

Closs J (1988) Assessment of sleep in hospital: a review of methods. *Journal of Advanced Nursing*, **13**, 501–510.

Cook R (1991) Plain speaking. *Nursing Times*, **87**, 19, 42.

Deberry S, Davis S and Reinhard K (1989) A comparison of meditation–relaxation and cognitive/behavioural techniques for reducing anxiety and depression in a geriatric population. *Journal of Geriatric Psychiatry*, **22**, 2, 231–247.

Ersser S (1988) Nursing beds and nursing therapy, In Pearson A (ed.) *Primary Nursing: Nursing in the Burford and Oxford Nursing Development Units*. London: Croom Helm.

Fordham M (1986) Sleep and rest. In Redfern S J (ed.) *Nursing Elderly People*. Edinburgh: Churchill Livingstone.

Finn E (1985) Still night silent night. *Nursing Mirror*, **160**, 2, 22.

Gomez G E and Gomez E A (1990) The special concerns of neuroleptic use in the elderly. *Journal of Psychosocial Nursing*, **28**, 1, 7–14.

Goodwin H (1988) Reflex zone therapy. In Rankin-Box D (ed.) *Complementary Health Therapies: a guide for nurses and the caring profession*. London: Croom Helm.

Gournay K (1988) Sleeping without drugs. *Nursing Times*, **84** 11, 46–49.

Husband L (1988) Therapeutic touch: a basis for excellence. In Johnson R A (ed.) *Recent Advances in Nursing*. Edinburgh: Churchill Livingstone.

Jackson S (1977) *Massage Therapy. A Holistic Way to Physical and Mental Wellbeing*. Wellingborough: Thorson Press.

Kearns S (1989) Insomnia in the Elderly. *Nursing Times*, **85**, 47, 32–33.

McMahon R (1990) Sleep therapies. *Surgical Nurse*, **3**, 5, 17–20.

McMahon R (1990) Sleep management. *Surgical Nurse*, **3**, 4, 25–27.

Morgan K, Healey D W and Healey P J (1989) Factors influencing persistent subjective insomnia in old age: a follow up study of good and poor sleepers aged 65 to 74. *Age and Ageing*, **18**, 117–122.

Norman L (1988) *The Reflexology Handbook*. London: Guild Publishing.

Ogilvie A J (1980) Sources and levels of noise on the ward at night. *Nursing Times*, **13**, 63, 6.

Oswald I (1984) Good, poor and disordered sleep. In Priest R G (ed.) *Sleep: An International Monograph*, 18–24. London: Update Books.

Passant H (1988) Aromatherapy on the wards. *International Journal of Aromatherapy*, **1**, 2, 8.

Pearson A (1988) *Primary Nursing: Nursing in the Burford and Oxford Nursing Development Units*. London: Croom Helm.

Rankin-Box D (1988) *Complementary Health Therapies: A Guide for Nurses and the Caring Profession*. London: Croom Helm.

Sims S (1986) Slow stroke back massage for cancer patients. *Nursing Times*, **82**, 47, 47–50.

Stead, W (1985) One awake all awake. *Nursing Mirror*, **160**, 16, 20–21.

Stokes G (1986) *Wandering*, Bicester: Winslow Press.

Sweeney S. (1978) Relaxation. In Carlson C and Blackwell R (eds) *Behavioural Concepts and Nursing Interventions* (2nd edn) Philadelphia: J B Lippincott.

Thomas M (1989) Fancy footwork. *Nursing Times*, **85**, 41, 42–44.

Tisserand R (1988) *Aromatherapy for Everyone*. London: Penguin.

Torrance (1990) Sleep and wound healing. *Surgical Nurse*, **3**, 2, 12–14.

Turton P (1989) Touch me, feel me, heal me. *Nursing Times*, **85**, 19, 42–44.

Valnet J (1980) *The Practice of Aromatherapy*. Essex: C W Daniel.

Walsh M and Ford P (1989) *Nursing Rituals: research and rational actions*. London: Heinemann.

Webster R (1986) Sleep in hospital. *Journal of Advanced Nursing*, **11**, 447–457.

Willis J (1989) A good night's sleep. *Nursing Times*, **85**, 47, 29–30.

Wise R (1989) Flower power. *Nursing Times*, **85**, 22, 45–47.

Wright S (1990) Selling out. *Nursing Standard*, **4**, 15, 46.

Zahourek R P (1988) *Relaxation and Imagery: Tools for Therapeutic Communication and Intervention*. Philadelphia: W B Saunders.

Chapter 5
Sleep and Pharmacology
Joanne A Blake

Introduction

We all attach a great deal of importance to a good night's sleep. It is one of the major factors with which we judge our personal well-being regardless of our age, sex or race. It is small wonder then that many people who suffer from insomnia or who experience sleeplessness on a reasonably frequent basis turn to drugs to relieve this problem. Clearly however, the achievement of sleep without the use of medication is the ideal and as Grahame and Aronson (1984) point out, there is no drug at present which can actually cure insomnia or induce 'normal' sleep.

Studies show that sleeping tablets (generally termed 'hypnotics') are some of the most extensively prescribed drugs, and that the use of these is related to age. Spiegel (1985) found that there is an increasing use of hypnotics throughout adult life well into the eighth decade, with a particularly sharp rise in use during middle age. It has been estimated that nearly a million elderly people take an hypnotic every night, despite the recommendation of the 1980 Committee on the Review of Medicines that they should only be prescribed for short-term use. Similarly, when researchers looked at patients over the age of 65 years being cared for by general practitioners, they found that more than 16% took hypnotics and that a quarter of occasional users had been taking them for over ten years. They also found a greater consumption among women than men (Morgan et al 1988).

Whilst there is a place for hypnotics in the treatment of insomnia, the adverse effects of tolerance, dependence and withdrawal difficulties are bringing their widespread use into question, and the emerging emphasis on the nurse as a health promoter makes the role of the practising nurse at night of crucial importance when the well-being of the patient is at stake.

Hypnotic Drug Usage in Hospital

People face particular sleep-related problems when they are admitted to hospital. For example, the strange environment, noise and stress all inhibit sleep. Every individual has their own habits with regard to sleep and rest.

However, these are 'vulnerable to manipulation by the constraints of the hospital philosophy and routine' (Webster and Thompson 1986). As a result many people who have never taken hypnotic drugs are prescribed and given them in hospital. This may be sensible in many cases, but it should not be an automatic process. Indeed, the British National Formulary (1989) advises that hypnotics should not be prescribed indiscriminately, and warns that in particular routine prescribing of these drugs in hospital is undesirable.

Night sedation is often prescribed to be taken as necessary (PRN) and it is nurses who are faced with the decision as to whether or not to administer the drug (Clapin-French 1986). Barnes (1968) suggested that sleeping tablets are often given to patients to relieve the nurse's frustration over a wakeful patient, rather than to help the patient to sleep. Other causative factors in the recurring pattern of over-medication may be inadequate staffing levels and other economic considerations.

However, these are not valid reasons for administering night sedation, and it requires an educational initiative for both staff and patients if an appropriate use of hypnotics is to be achieved.

This chapter aims to provide the information supported by research to facilitate the knowledgeable and appropriate administration of these drugs by nurses, and to enable them to advise their patients wisely on the advantages and disadvantages of using hypnotic drug therapy.

The History of Hypnotic Drugs

For centuries people have been discovering and using natural substances to induce sleep, such as derivatives from poppies and herbs. In the 19th century chemists began the search for a suitable synthetic alternative, with the first hypnotic drugs being marketed towards the end of the century. One of the first of these drugs was chloral hydrate, which along with its derivatives such as dichloralphenazone is still widely used today (Morgan 1987). In the early 20th century barbiturates such as amylobarbitone were introduced as hypnotics and tranquillisers, and they rapidly gained in popularity. However, they were soon found to have two major faults: firstly, they were very addictive, and secondly, they were frequently fatal if taken in an overdose.

Since the 1960s the group of drugs called the benzodiazepines has gradually replaced the barbiturates as the main hypnotic and anxiolytic agents of today. Even though the benzodiazepines are generally safer than the barbiturates in that even a large overdose is rarely fatal, they still have many problems attached to their use.

There is a slow but increasing movement away from the casual prescription of hypnotic drugs which occurred in the sixties and seventies, with a growing realisation that they should be used only when a clearly defined reason can be identified, and that their use should be constantly monitored.

Reasons for Using Hypnotics

Nicholson (1986) suggested three reasons for using hypnotics:

1. To shorten sleep onset for people who are experiencing difficulty in getting off to sleep
2. To reduce night-time wakefulness
3. To provide an anxiolytic effect during the next day for an individual who may be experiencing a degree of anxiety as well as insomnia.

He goes on to suggest that hypnotics are most appropriately used in the short term with patients whose insomnia has developed recently, and that their use in chronic insomnia is unwise.

Insomnia is a highly subjective symptom which is based on whether the individual *feels* that they have not slept well (Goldson 1981). In nursing there are many occasions when patients have complained that they have slept poorly, but that the perception of the nursing staff is that they have slept soundly for long periods. Before making a decision about how to treat a patient with insomnia therefore, it is important to make an assessment of their sleep disorder and possibly classify it into one of the following types.

Short-Term Insomnia   This may be caused by an emotional disturbance or serious illness and may last for a few weeks. In general, the use of hypnotics for people who have an emotional cause, such as a bereavement, should be avoided as this can easily slide into long-term reliance (Lader 1986). Only if all alternative methods fail should a low-dose hypnotic be prescribed, and this should be used intermittently over a week or two. Lader suggests that the patient is advised to try to get to sleep without the medication for an hour or so before resorting to the sleeping tablet.

Transient Insomnia   This occurs when the normal sleep-wake cycle is disturbed due to circumstances such as jet-lag or shiftwork. Treatment with benzodiazepines may be useful in helping an individual get off to sleep during these irregular times. A low-dose, short-acting drug is most appropriate in order to avoid sleepiness or other residual effects the next day.

Chronic Insomnia   The three most common causes of insomnia are anxiety, depression and pain (Smith 1985). Unfortunately people are often prescribed a hypnotic drug instead of the underlying cause of the insomnia being properly assessed and treated. A study in Ulster (Irwin and Cupples 1986) found that 65% of patients presenting with psychiatric, psychological or social problems had been prescribed drugs.

Where the patient is experiencing sleeplessness as a result of anxiety, which is characterised by a difficulty getting off to sleep, alternative methods such as those described in Chapter 4 are a better choice of management than hypnotics. If the patient is depressed, he will often experience the effect of early morning waking, with proper management of the depression being preferable to the use of sleeping tablets. If the use of an anti-depressant is indicated, then drugs such as Mianserin will help to alleviate the depression and also promote sleep through its mild sedative effect.

People who are addicted to drugs or alcohol also commonly suffer with chronic insomnia. Usually the problem resolves once the person has overcome the addiction, however it can persist for several months. Hypnotics should be avoided in the treatment of such insomnia, as substance abusers will rapidly become dependent on those also (Lennane and Tuck 1989).

Other physical causes of chronic insomnia include restless leg syndrome and muscular jerking of the legs at night (nocturnal myoclonus), both of which may prevent the patient from getting off to sleep. These aggravating conditions are sometimes treated with hypnotics which only reduce the awareness of these leg movements rather than actually lessening their occurrence.

Ageing and Insomnia

Older people are the most frequent users of over-the-counter hypnotic treatments (Clapin-French 1986). The normal ageing process changes individuals' sleep patterns, so that as they get older their sleep tends to get more fragmented over a 24-hour period, with catnaps during the day being commonplace. However, many elderly people still expect a good eight hours' sleep each night and conclude that they have a sleep problem when this does not occur. Elderly people also have an increased incidence of depression and are more vulnerable to physical illnesses which may cause pain and discomfort, or other sleep disturbing symptoms such as nocturia. Despite all these valid reasons for older people to turn to sleeping tablets for relief of their insomnia, health workers need to be vigilant as to the appropriateness of their use as the elderly are more susceptible to the adverse effects of hypnotic drugs.

The Benzodiazepines as Hypnotics

The benzodiazepines can cause considerable changes in the different stages of sleep, although there is little evidence of this having a harmful effect. These drugs reduce the amount of rapid eye movement sleep (Morgan 1987), cause a decrease in slow wave sleep [Stages 3 and 4 (Roth et al 1982)], and a corresponding increase in light (Stage 2) sleep. Tissue and cell repair, growth, and recovery from fatigue are all associated with slow wave sleep, but there is no evidence that they are affected by its suppression through the use of benzodiazepines. Adam (1984) concluded that what happens is that the benzodiazepines affect the generation of the electrical waves of the brain without disturbing any of the associated biological processes.

The benzodiazepines have the effect of aiding the onset of sleep, reducing the number of wakenings during the night and increasing the overall amount of time spent asleep. They are not general depressants of the central nervous system, rather they appear to work through specific receptor sites in the brain membranes. The highest concentration of these sites is found in the cerebral cortical regions (Nimmo 1984a). These drugs also seem to function through specific receptor sites in the limbic system which is the area of the brain associated particularly with the emotions and feelings. These receptors contain an inhibitory neurotransmitter called gamma-aminobutyric acid (GABA) which is potentiated by the benzodiazepines. The resulting inhibition of the nervous system has the desired action of inducing sleep. The effect of benzodiazepines is increased by alcohol and other centrally acting drugs.

Benzodiazepines differ pharmacologically from one another and an understanding of these differences is needed in order to make an appropriate choice of drug. For instance, the rate of onset of action differs among these drugs; one that has a rapid onset is more appropriate for patients who have difficulty getting to sleep, whereas a slower onset tablet would be more suitable if the problem was waking early in the morning.

When comparing the benzodiazepines, it is necessary to consider their pharmokinetic properties with particular regard for their rates and methods of absorption, distribution, metabolism, elimination and consequently their duration of action.

Absorption

It is the rate at which a drug is absorbed which determines its rate of onset of action. The benzodiazepines are well absorbed from the gastro-intestinal tract and peak levels of the drug in the plasma are usually reached within 1–3 hours. Antacids can seriously interfere with their absorption, and as benzodiazepines should be taken on an empty stomach they should be taken before any such indigestion remedy (Hyman and Arana 1987).

Distribution and Elimination

All benzodiazepines penetrate the blood-brain barrier easily, which ensures the relatively rapid action that is required to make hypnotics effective in promoting sleep. As it is distributed around the body, the plasma concentration of the drug starts to fall. If the plasma concentration drops quickly during distribution then the duration of action of the drug may be short. The duration of action is also affected by the rate of elimination, but generally, the elimination phase is slower than the distribution phase (Nicholson 1982).

Metabolism

Some benzodiazepines such as flurazepam are metabolised in the liver to form metabolites which remain active and so extend the effect of the drug for a longer period of time. Other drugs, such as temazepam, conjugate in the liver with glucuronic acid and are excreted in the urine without forming active metabolites. Clearly liver function can be a major factor in the metabolism of the benzodiazepines, a particular point to consider if the patient has liver disease.

Duration of Action

As has been described, the duration of action of these drugs is determined by their rate of absorption, distribution, elimination and by whether they produce active metabolites. The duration of action is often described in terms of the drug's half-life, which is the time taken for the plasma concentration to be reduced by half. If an active metabolite is produced, it is the half-life of the metabolite which needs to be considered. It is important to be aware of the duration of action of the drugs that patients are prescribed, as this will indicate whether residual side-effects such as drowsiness or impaired performance will be experienced the next day.

Some people who take a benzodiazepine with a long half-life [such as nitrazepam which has an elimination half-life of 20–31 hours (Nimmo 1984a)] will experience an accumulation of the drug as one dose is not fully eliminated before the next dose is taken. Accumulation results in a greater build-up of tolerance to the drug and impaired performance during the day. By contrast, more rapidly eliminated benzodiazepines have a shorter duration of action and seem to be preferable. They cause less residual effects and less disturbance of rapid eye movement sleep, particularly when taken in small doses. However, problems do occur when a person stops taking them after a period of time in that they can suffer from a withdrawal phenomenon known as 'rebound insomnia', which will be discussed later in this chapter.

Tolerance

There are a number of different views regarding the development of tolerance to the benzodiazepines. The committee on the Review of Medicines (1980) concluded that most hypnotics lose their sleep promoting action in 3–14 days of continuous use. However, other reports suggest that the effectiveness is maintained for longer periods. For example, Oswald et al (1982) reported findings which indicated that nitrazepam is effective for up to 32 weeks. Whatever the exact speed of onset of tolerance may be, it is clear that benzodiazepines lose their effectiveness with regular use.

Types of Benzodiazepines

This category of drug can be broadly divided into two types: prolonged-acting and shorter-acting.

Prolonged-Acting Benzodiazepines

Nitrazepam and flurazepam belong to this category. They both have long elimination half-lives with the consequent problem of accumulation which causes problems the next day if the drug is taken every night. Marked impairment of psychomotor performance in elderly people has been observed after a single 10mg dose of nitrazepam (Goldson 1981). This type of benzodiazepine may be useful for people who awaken early or for use post-operatively when morning drowsiness may be beneficial. However, for elderly people and those who have to drive or operate machinery in the morning, use of these drugs can increase the risk of an accident.

Shorter-Acting Benzodiazepines

One of the more common shorter acting benzodiazepines is temazepam, which has a half life of 8–10 hours. This makes it relatively free from residual effects in the morning, although some patients who take a nightly dose of 20mg or more do seem to experience them. Lormetazepam is similar in action to temazepam but not so widely used. Loprazolam is also shorter acting but is more slowly absorbed making it less suitable for people who have difficulty getting to sleep.

Adverse Effects of the Benzodiazepines

Side-effects from benzodiazepines occur most frequently when high doses are taken over a prolonged period of time. Most of the side-effects are extensions of the therapeutic effects of the drugs, leading to drowsiness, tiredness, lethargy, vertigo, dizziness and particularly in the elderly, ataxia, confusion and impaired judgement. The British National Formulary (1989) indicates that individuals may also feel aggressive, excited, anxious and exhibit anti-social behaviour.

Impaired Psychomotor Performance

Goldson (1981) found that a single dose of nitrazepam 10mg can cause a marked impairment of psychomotor performance in elderly people for a period of 36 hours. Even in young people impaired judgement may persist for several hours after wakening leaving the individual more vulnerable to accidents. Adverse psychomotor effects may become progressively more apparent after a week or two of continuous treatment (Grahame-Smith and Aronson 1984). Hindmarch (1981) investigated the effects of benzodiazepines on psychomotor performance and found that the dose of drug taken was an important variable. Whilst significant effects were noted after nightly use of nitrazepam 10mg, the same effects were not apparent after taking 5mg nightly.

Such adverse effects may affect an individual's recovery in hospital. Regular night sedation may delay an individual's recovery from a cerebral vascular accident due to impaired day-time judgement, balance and co-ordination, and may contribute to the number of falls occurring in the elderly population.

Dependence

Benzodiazepines are the most common drugs for which repeat prescriptions are written. Long-term users of hypnotics are often reluctant to stop taking them, or even to change to a different one despite their general practitioner's recommendation. The development of dependence on these drugs may be the explanation for this. Individuals are afraid that if they stop taking their regular tablets, the quality of their sleep might deteriorate. They may have also heard of people who have had bad withdrawal symptoms. Therefore, the benzodiazepines may induce both physical and psychological dependence on their use (Lader 1981).

Habits and routines can make people feel secure and, as Morgan (1987) points out, the taking of a hypnotic can easily become part of a bed-time routine. A person who has 'got in the habit' of taking a drug in order for him to achieve what he perceives to be a satisfactory level of sleep can be said to be psychologically dependent, whereas if a person continues to take a benzodiazepine so as to avoid certain unpleasant withdrawal symptoms then he is physically dependent. Both of these types can occur in anyone taking these drugs, however the risk of dependence is higher when the drug has been taken regularly for longer than two months (Grahame-Smith and Aronson 1984).

Rebound Insomnia

Long-term users who abruptly stop taking benzodiazepines are most at risk of suffering from withdrawal symptoms such as anxiety, apprehension, tremor, nausea, vomiting and insomnia (Committee on the Review of Medicines 1980). The degree to which these symptoms occur can vary from mild to completely debilitating.

Users of the short-acting benzodiazepines are particularly vulnerable to rebound insomnia. Rebound is a general phenomenon which occurs on the withdrawal of drugs that affect the central nervous system (CNS) (Wood and Rue 1982). During the time when the drug is being taken, the CNS changes in an attempt to counteract the drug. When the medication is abruptly withdrawn, the counteracting mechanism is still operating, resulting in effects which are opposite to those of the drug. Therefore the withdrawal of a benzodiazepine leads to a rebound effect of insomnia and anxiety. Rebound insomnia can occur after only one week of treatment on a short-acting benzodiazepine. The longer-acting varieties tend to cause less acute effects on withdrawal as they have longer elimination half-lives. This causes a percentage of the drug to remain in the body and be excreted slowly, resulting in a gradual drop in the plasma level which diminishes the effects of the withdrawal.

The very short-acting benzodiazepine, triazolam, which was withdrawn from use in Great Britain by the Committee on the Safety of Medicines in 1991, was found to have particular rebound problems. The drug had such a short half-life that it was almost completely eliminated long before the next dose was taken, resulting in withdrawal effects occurring during the day. Morgan and Oswald (1982) found that this may cause rebound anxiety, with some individuals experiencing increased levels of worry and agitation during the day. Other side-effects of triazolam which led to the ban included depression and memory loss.

Gillen et al (1989) reviewed recent studies which have looked at the occurrence of rebound insomnia in individuals taking triazolam, temazepam and flurazepam. The side-effect was found to be common after withdrawing from triazolam 0.5mg, but less so after 0.25mg. The rebound effect took the form of a reduction in the total amount of time asleep, an increase in the time taken to get to sleep and a feeling that sleep was not effective. They also found some, but not a significant amount of, rebound effects after withdrawal from temazepam (15–30mg). Flurazepam (15–30mg), which is a prolonged acting benzodiazepine, showed no rebound effects during the first three nights post-withdrawal but mild effects were experienced during nights 4–10 as the drug level in the plasma reduced.

Withdrawal Methods

In order to avoid withdrawal symptoms, users of benzodiazepines need to gradually taper off the dose of the drug being taken. Professional support and guidance may be needed during withdrawal, particularly for long-term users who have developed dependence.

Ellis (1988) suggests a four-pronged approach for weaning people off tablets, which involves the use of honesty, planning, a gradual approach and reward. A tapering regime can be worked out jointly between the individual and the doctor, which may involve reducing the dose week by week and trying to use the benzodiazepine only when the individual feels most in need of it. Advice is required on alternative ways of promoting sleep and also on what factors inhibit sleep, such as evening coffee-drinking.

In a hospital setting, some patients are prescribed sleeping tablets to take home on discharge even though they only started taking them whilst they were an in-patient. This can precipitate long-term use, especially if the patient is able to receive repeat prescriptions easily from the general practitioner. This may be perceived by the patient as an indication from the doctor that he now needs the drug and psychological dependence may develop. Attempts should normally be made to withdraw such temporary users from their sleeping tablets before discharge. In contrast, a hospital admission may also provide a valuable opportunity to review long-term use of benzodiazepines. With professional support and encouragement, a long-term user may be able to decrease the dosage and frequency of use, transfer on to a short-acting drug, or even stop taking benzodiazepines altogether.

The Non-Benzodiazepine Hypnotics

As the benzodiazepines are the most commonly used drugs for night sedation, they have been discussed in some detail in this chapter. There are however other drugs which are used on a regular basis and their use is worthy of exploration.

Chloral Hydrate

Chloral hydrate was formulated in 1832 and was one of the first hypnotics used. Along with its more widely used derivatives dichloralphenazone and triclofos sodium, it is still in use today. Chloral hydrate is metabolised in the liver, forming an active metabolite which has an elimination half-life of 8–10 hours. Another metabolite is also formed which has a half-life of about four days (Nimmo 1984a). Therefore if a person takes chloral hydrate every night, they will be at risk of the effects of accumulation, including day-time drowsiness and impaired psychomotor performance.

A common side-effect is gastric irritation, therefore the drug is administered as a liquid or in capsule form to reduce this effect. Other side effects include over-excitement and delirium. Sudden withdrawal of the drug should be avoided as that too can cause delirium.

Chlormethiazole

This drug is used in particular as a hypnotic for the treatment of insomnia in the elderly. It has an elimination half-life of 7–8 hours and does not appear to have any cumulative hangover effects. Lilenberg et al (1986) studied the effects of chlormethiazole when taken for five nights by elderly volunteers. They reported that the subjects went to sleep more quickly, awoke less often and felt that their sleep was generally slightly improved. From electroencephalograph readings, there seemed to be no disruption to the progression of the stages of sleep, and no rebound insomnia or impaired psychomotor performance was observed.

Dependence on chlormethiazole has been noted to occur and, as with all hypnotics, its use should be restricted to low doses over a short period only. Other side-effects include conjunctival irritation, tingling in the nose and sneezing (Nimmo 1984a).

Promethazine

In the unusual circumstances of a child needing night sedation the drug of choice is promethazine. Hypnotics should only be used for children in the treatment of night terrors and sleep walking. The British National Formulary (1989) states that any other use cannot be justified.

Inhibitors of Sleep

Coffee and Caffeine

Most people are aware that coffee contains caffeine which is a stimulant also found in colas and some analgesics. Coffee has been found to produce sleep disturbances (Goldstein 1965, Brezinova 1974) which include a reduction in time spent asleep, an increase in the time taken to get to sleep, and an increase in the number of awakenings.

Karacan et al (1976) studied the effects of different doses of coffee and caffeine on the sleep of young adults. The equivalent of a cup of coffee (1.1mg caffeine per 1kg body weight) taken half an hour before bed-time had little or no effect on their sleep. However, the eqivalent of two cups radically affected the volunteers' ability to get to sleep. They also reported lack of satisfaction in the quality of their sleep. The four-cup equivalent taken half an hour before retiring affected all stages of sleep. The total amount of rapid-eye-movement sleep was increased and was concentrated in the early part of the night. The same people were also given a four-cup equivalent dose of decaffeinated coffee which produced no effect on their sleep.

Coffee should therefore be regarded as a potential cause of insomnia, and the consumption of coffee within a few hours of bed-time is best avoided.

Tea

Tea has also been a subject of interest with regard to sleep problems, being both a stimulant and a diuretic. Its stimulant properties can cause difficulty getting off to sleep and its diuretic effects can cause nocturnal wakenings. In a study of elderly people (Morgan et al 1989), poor sleepers were found to report significantly higher levels of tea consumption than the good sleepers.

Alcohol

Small quantities of alcohol have a soporific effect and may aid the onset of sleep. However, alcohol has been found to cause more awakenings during the night and changes in the duration of the various stages of sleep (Williams et al 1983). In particular alcohol may abolish rapid-eye-movement sleep and there is a rebound effect if the person withdraws from the alcohol, including nightmares and insomnia for a few weeks.

Pharmacological Inhibitors of Sleep

Nurses need to be familiar with the nature of the drugs being used in the treatment of patients in their care. If a patient is prescribed a drug which is known to cause insomnia, it may be appropriate to share this information with him. Both nurse and patient would then be aware of the potential problem and plan care accordingly.

Beta-blockers are known to cause sleep disturbances. The more water-soluble ones, such as atenolol and nadolol, cause less disturbance than the lipid soluble ones as they are less likely to cross the blood-brain barrier (British National Formulary 1989). Propranolol can cause central nervous system side-effects including vivid nightmares and sleep disturbances (Nimmo 1984b). The anti-hypertensive drug methyldopa has been found to cause insomnia, both during treatment with the drug and on withdrawal (Davies 1981).

Jahanshahi (1986) reports that amphetamines reduce sleep duration and suppress rapid-eye-movement sleep, causing a rebound effect on cessation of treatment. Drugs used to treat Parkinson's disease, such as levadopa and amantadine hydrochloride, can cause insomnia, as can Ephedrine which is commonly used for reversible airways obstruction. Similarly, treatment with aminophylline and theophylline may also lead to sleep disturbances.

Conclusion

This chapter has explored the use and misuse of hypnotic drug therapy. It can be clearly seen that hypnotics have a place in the short-term treatment of sleep disturbances, particularly for transient insomnia. However, the use of hypnotics must be balanced against the knowledge of adverse effects: impaired psychomotor performance, accumulative residual effects, dependence, rebound insomnia and other withdrawal difficulties. Clear note needs to be taken of the recommendations that hypnotics should only be used for short periods, in low dosage and, where possible, intermittently.

Proper assessment and treatment of the *cause* of sleep disturbance is essential, as opposed to routine treatment of the symptom of insomnia with hypnotics which may be inappropriate. With a deeper understanding of the nature of sleep, the drugs used to promote sleep and those which can inhibit it, nurses will be able to assess and plan care, advise patients and monitor drug therapy more knowledgeably.

References

Adam K (1984) Are poor sleepers changed into good sleepers by hypnotic drugs? In Hindmarch I, Ott H and Roth T (eds) *Sleep. Benzodiazepines and Performance.* Berlin: Springer-Verlag.

Barnes E (1968) *Psychosocial Nursing. Studies from the Cassel Hospital, London.* London: Tavistock.

Brezinova V (1974) Effects of caffeine on sleep: EEG study in late middle age people. *British Journal of Clinical Pharmacology*, **1**, 203–208.

British National Formulary (1989) 17. London: British Medical Association and Royal Pharmaceutical Society of Great Britain.

Clapin-French E (1986) Sleep patterns of aged persons in long-term care facilities. *Journal of Advanced Nursing*, **11**, 57–66.

Committee on the Review of Medicines (1980) Systematic review of benzodiazepines. *British Medical Journal*, **280**, 910–912.

Davies D M (1981) *Textbook of Adverse Drug Reactions* (2nd edn). Oxford: Oxford University Press.

Ellis P (1988) A four-pronged approach for weaning patients off tablets. *Geriatric Medicine*, **18**, 7, 49–52.

Gillin J C, Spinweber C L and Johnson L C (1989) Rebound insomnia: a critical review. *Journal of Clinical Psychopharmacology*, **9**, 3, 161–172.

Goldstein A, Warren R and Kaizer S (1965) Psychotropic effects of caffeine in man. 1: Individual differences in sensitivity to caffeine-induced wakefulness. *Journal of Pharmacology*, **149**, 156–159.

Goldson R L (1981) Management of sleep disorders in the elderly. *Current Therapeutics*, **22**, 59–67.

Grahame-Smith D G and Aronson J K (1984) *Oxford Textbook of Clinical Pharmacology and Drug Therapy*. Oxford: Oxford University Press.

Hindmarch I (1981) Psychotropic drugs and psychomotor performance. In Murray R, Ghodse H, Harris C, Williams D and Williams P (eds). *The Misuse of Psychotropic Drugs*. London: Gaskell.

Hyman S E and Arana G W (1987) *Handbook of Psychiatric Drug Therapy*. Boston/ Toronto: Little, Brown and Company.

Irwin W G and Cupples M E (1986) *Journal of Royal College of General Practitioners*, **36**, 366–368.

Jahanshahi M (1986) Insomnia. *Nursing*, **3**, 9, 328–332.

Karacan I, Thornby J I, Anch H M, Booth G H, Williams R L and Salis P J (1976) Dose-related sleep disturbances induced by coffee and caffeine. *Clinical Pharmacology and Therapeutics*, **20**, 6, 682–689.

Kales A, Soldatos C R, Bixter E O and Kales J D (1983) Rebound insomnia and rebound anxiety: a review. *Pharmacology*, **26**, 3, 121–137.

Lader M (1981) Benzodiazepine dependence. In Murray R, Ghodse H, Harris C, Williams D and Williams P (eds). *The Misuse of Psychotropic Drugs*. London: Gaskell.

Lader M (1986) A practical guide to prescribing hypnotic benzodiazepines. *British Medical Journal*, **293**, 1048–1049.

Lennane K J and Tuck R T (1989) Neurological and psychiatric aspects of alcoholism. *Medicine International*, February, 2557–2561.

Liljenberg B and Almqvist M (1986) The effects of chlormethiazole in EEG. Recorded sleep in normal elderly volunteers. *Acta Psychiatrica Scandinavia*, **329**, 73, 34–39.

Morgan K and Oswald I (1982) Anxiety caused by a short-life hypnotic. *British Medical Journal* (Clinical Research), **284**, 942.

Morgan K (1987) *Sleep and Ageing*. London: Croom Helm.

Morgan K, Dallosse H, Erbrahim S, Arie T and Fentem P H (1988) Prevalence, frequency and duration of hypnotic drug use amongst the elderly living at home. *British Medical Journal*, **296**, 601–602.

Morgan K, Healey D W and Healey P J (1989) Factors influencing persistent subjective insomnia in old age: a follow-up study of good and poor sleepers aged 65–74, *Age and Ageing*, **18**, 117–122.

Nicholson A N (1982) Hypnotics: their place in therapeutics. *Drugs*, **31**, 164–176.

Nimmo W S (1984a) Hypnotics, sedatives, tranquillisers and antidepressants. In Girdwood R H (ed.) *Clinical Pharmacology*. London: Bailliere Tindall.

Nimmo J (1984b) Drugs acting on the cardiovascular system. In Girdwood R H (ed.) *Clinical Pharmacology*. London: Bailliere Tindall.

Oswald I, French C, Adam D and Gilham J (1982) Benzodiazepine hypnotics remain effective for 24 weeks. *British Medical Journal*, **284**, 860–863.

Roth T, Zorick F, Wittig R and Roehrs T (1982) Pharmacological and medical considerations in hypnotic use. *Sleep*, **5**, 546–552.

Smith S (1985) Drugs and sleep. *Nursing Times*, **81**, 6, 36–37.

Spiegel R (1985) Sleep and its disorders. In Pathy M S J (ed.) *Principles and Practice of Geriatric Medicine*. Chichester: John Wiley and Sons.

Swift C G (1986) Special problems relating to the use of hypnotics in the elderly. *Acta Psychiatrica Scandinavia*, **329**, 73, 92–98.

Sykes J B (ed.) (1982) *The Concise Oxford Dictionary of Current English* (7th edn). Oxford: Clarendon Press.

Webster R A and Thompson D R (1986) Sleep in hospital. *Journal of Advanced Nursing*, **11**, 447–457.

Williams D L, McLean A W and Cairns J (1983) Dose-related effects of ethanol on the sleep of young women. *Journal of Studies on Alcohol*, **44**, 515–523.

Wood C and Rue Y (1982) Experience with triazolobenzodiazepines as hypnotics. *The Royal Society of Medicine Forum Series*, 8.

Chapter 6
Assessment and Control of Post-operative Pain at Night
S José Closs

'I fear the nights most of all, I try and get a grip on myself but the dark presses in on me and there seems no escape from the pain.'

From Raiman (1986)

Introduction

Pain and difficulties with sleep are two of the more unpleasant experiences commonly faced by surgical patients during their stay in hospital. Pain may have a particularly negative effect on sleep, in some cases preventing it completely, for one or more nights. Dealing with these patients' problems is an essential part of nursing in many clinical areas, not only in surgical wards. Problems of sleeping and controlling pain cannot be considered in isolation from all the other factors which are likely to impinge on the hospitalised patient, or indeed, from each other. There are, however, some relatively underexploited ways in which nurses may help patients to manage their pain at night.

The first part of this chapter is concerned with why it is important for hospital patients to have their pain well controlled and why they should sleep well. Then there is a discussion of pain at night and the difficulties inherent in its assessment. The remainder of the chapter outlines some possibilities for helping patients to manage their pain, thereby improving their ability to sleep.

Why Post-operative Patients Need Sleep

Research literature suggests that there are three main reasons why patients should be helped to sleep adequately. First, sleep appears to have a role in physical restoration; second, sleep deprivation has detrimental effects on mood and performance; and third, in theory at least, beliefs about sleep may have a tangible effect on health.

Sleep and Physical Restoration

Tissue building processes are most active during sleep. These anabolic activities include protein synthesis and cell division, each of which is required for wound healing (see for example Fisher 1968, Valk and Van den Bosch 1979, Clausen et al 1979). Hormones are involved in the regulation of healing processes too. For example, catabolic hormones such as catecholamines and cortisol inhibit protein synthesis and these are reduced during sleep (Akerstedt and Froberg 1979, Weitzman et al 1983). Growth hormone (GH) is secreted mostly during deep (slow wave) sleep. This hormone is involved in amino acid uptake and protein synthesis. Together these pieces of evidence point to the conclusion that physical healing is promoted by sleep.

Sleep and Psychological State

The psychological consequences of disturbed sleep are well documented. Horne (1983) discussed changes in the functioning of the central nervous system (CNS) after two or more nights of total deprivation. These included 'behavioural irritability, suspiciousness, speech slurring [and] minor visual misperceptions'. Recovery from surgery depends on the patient co-operating with nursing staff in efforts to eat, drink, mobilise and so on, and negative mood states may interfere with these activities. The effect of sleep on mood was investigated by Shaver et al (1989) who studied 71 healthy women and found that sleep had a positive effect on mood state. Their suggestion that this finding provided a rationale for promoting nursing interventions designed to help patients improve their sleep seems very reasonable.

Beliefs and Health

The effects of belief on health are currently receiving some considerable attention. There are increasing numbers of research studies which have investigated how the mind converts ideas and expectations into biological realities. Although there is little information available specifically on the effects of sleep beliefs on health, several studies have produced convincing results concerning the placebo effect and the power of suggestion.

Patients who were told that they were going to have spinal anaesthetics and would therefore experience post-operative headaches were told at the last minute that they would actually receive general anaesthesia (Katz 1977). Even so, they still suffered 'classical examples of spinal anaesthesia headache'. An interesting example of the placebo effect was shown by Fielding et al (1983). Patients undergoing chemotherapy were told that they would lose their hair as a result. One-third of them received a placebo instead, but they still lost their hair. Obviously some beliefs can have a powerful influence on biological outcomes, and there is no reason to suppose that beliefs about sleep do not. Although there are bound to be considerable individual variations in such beliefs, for at least some of those people who believe that poor sleep results in ill health, it may in fact do so.

Sleep appears to be important to the individual in various ways then, some physiological, some psychological and some a combination of the two. Evidently the promotion of sleep should be a high priority for nurses caring for patients at night.

Why Post-operative Patients Don't Need Pain

Freedom from severe pain of any kind should be a basic human right. While acute pain usually has a protective effect, for example by immobilising a broken limb, it also may have detrimental effects on various body systems. These may be particularly problematic to the post-operative patient. Pain can reduce mobility, exacerbate nervous, metabolic and hormonal disruption, increase the possibiliy of long-term pain and cause disrupted sleep.

Effects of Reduced Mobility Due to Pain

Reduced mobility can produce a series of familiar post-operative complications. These include deep vein thrombosis, damage to pressure areas, reluctance to mobilise compounded by the resulting muscle atrophy, and in some cases reduced respiratory movements leading to hypoxia and respiratory tract infection (see Bonica 1990). Pain contributes to the development of all these problems which are obviously best avoided.

Pain-induced Nervous, Hormonal and Metabolic Changes

Sympathetic nervous activity and circulating catecholamines both increase during acute pain. These changes may result in raised heart rate and blood pressure with the possibility of ischaemia of the myocardium and other tissues. Tissue breakdown is a normal result of surgery, when anabolic hormones such as cortisol and ACTH promote the breakdown of proteins and the mobilisation of free fatty acids (Nimmo and Duthie 1987). Pain increases this response, accelerating catabolic processes when tissue restoration is most desirable. Bladder functions may also be affected: persistent post-operative pain can lead to a reduction in the motility of the urethra and bladder so that passing urine becomes more difficult and infection of the urinary tract becomes more likely (Bonica and Benedetti 1980). Further, visceral pain-induced sympathetic hyperactivity has been shown to inhibit gastrointestinal activity producing ileus, nausea and vomiting (Bing 1936).

Prolonged Post-operative Pain

The stimulation of the CNS during surgical trauma can result in prolonged hyperexcitability of the CNS. This sensitisation changes the perceptions of sensations, so tht stimuli that should be innocuous, feel painful (Woolf 1983). Not only that, but it may be months before this returns to normal and the painful response subsides. This sensitisation can be prevented by giving opioid drugs before, during and after surgery. Failure to control this priming of the CNS during the perioperative period can lead to long-term pain (Bach et al 1988).

The Effects of Pain on Sleep

Most importantly in the context of controlling pain at night, the effects of pain on sleep can be severe. Animal research (Carli et al 1987) has shown that persistent pain shortens sleeping time by repeatedly interrupting sleep and reducing both restorative slow wave sleep and dreaming sleep. A few studies have investigated the association between the sleep and pain of hospital inpatients. A small but seminal study of 37 medical patients (Marks and Sachar 1973) showed that for three-quarters of them sleep was the physical function most often interfered with by pain. Intensive care patients were the subjects of a study by Jones et al (1979), and for them pain was a significant factor in sleep loss. In 1983 Sriwatanakul and others interviewed 81 post-operative patients and found that 56.7% of them expressed some level of distress at the effect of pain on their sleep. Seers (1987) found that almost two-thirds of a sample of 67 patients were disturbed by pain on their first post-operative night. More recently Closs (1988, 1991) found that post-operative patients cited pain and discomfort as the factors which disturbed their sleep more than any other. Pain evidently has a profoundly negative effect on sleep for many surgical patients.

Donovan et al (1987) conducted a larger study of 353 patients, and found that sleep was one of four major factors perceived as decreasing pain. These findings were corroborated by a survey of 100 post-operative patients (Closs 1991). One-third of them felt that a good night's sleep reduced pain intensity and three-quarters felt that sleep helped them to cope more effectively with their pain.

These observations suggest that patients feel that pain and sleep are linked in various ways: while pain disturbs sleep, sleep reduces pain intensity and increases the ability to cope with pain.

Patients' Experiences of Pain at Night

Circadian (circa=about, dies=a day) rhythms have been noted for particular kinds of pain. Biliary colic typically begins during the night and tends to recur at the same clock time (Rigas et al 1990). Gobel and Cordes (1990) found that sensitivity to intense headache was greatest at 2am and least at 2pm. Twenty-four hour fluctuations in post-operative pain are less clear, although Pollman and Hildebrandt (1987) found that following dental surgery the greatest number of doses of analgesics were given around 6am on the second and third post-operative days. An interesting piece of research by Burns et al (1989) recorded the patterns of self-administration of morphine among post-operative patients. A circadian fluctuation was noted, with peak requirements at around 9am and 8pm. This latter finding was corroborated by Closs (1991) who found that maximum numbers of doses of 'on demand' opioids were given between 8am–12pm and 8pm–12am. Although some kinds of pain are worse during the night, analgesic consumption appears to be greatest early in the morning and mid-evening. Even so, this does not mean that surgical patients are pain free during the night.

Examination of the medication charts of post-operative patients showed that they received roughly half as many doses of analgesics at night than during the day (Closs 1990, 1991). Since almost half of the patients in the second of these studies felt that pain was worse at night than during the day, it appears that the assessment and treatment of pain at night presents something of a problem. This observation was borne out by patients' comments on their experiences of night-time pain:

'It's more intense in the middle of the night, basically because you're tired and feel on your own.'

'The pain does seem worse at night. There's nothing worse than having pain and watching the clock go round. You close your eyes at 4.20 and open them at 4.25 – it's terrible.'

'All pain gets worse at night. . . . It seems to flare up during the night and ease off around 9am, even though you don't have a painkiller.'

'It's terrible at night – it gives you nightmares if you can sleep at all. There's nothing to think about except the pain.'

(Closs 1991)

How Can Nurses Help Patients at Night?

Nurses can only help patients who suffer pain if they make accurate and timely assessments of their pain, followed by the appropriate provision of analgesics and/or other complementary methods of pain control. It is essential that this should then be followed by monitoring the effectiveness of any intervention used. This is an area of care requiring some careful empirical research into the problems specific to night-time pain control.

Difficulties of Assessing Pain at Night

Patients have a wide range of ways of expressing pain, including vocal behaviour and non-vocal expression. It is highly likely that patients become more inhibited about overtly expressing their pain at night. Although there is considerable research into nurses' preferred methods of assessment and their frequent inadequacy, little information is available on the specific difficulties encountered at night.

Craig and Prkachin (1983) described a variety of potential expressions of painful distress (Table 6.1).

Table 6.1 Potential expressions of painful distress

Vocal behaviour	
Language:	complaint, appeals, qualitative description, ratings, demands, exclamations
Paralinguistic vocalisations:	crying, screaming, moaning, sighing
Non-vocal expression	
Facial:	distortion, grimacing, specific configurations
Limbs:	startle, withdrawal reflexes, clutching or rubbing painful area, locomotor activity
Postural:	guarded or unusual postures, inactivity
Autonomic activity:	blanching, flushing, panting, vomiting

Patients are asked to indicate which option best describes their pain. The number of categories of pain description vary, as do the descriptors themselves, depending on which particular scale is selected for use. It is likely that the simpler scales are the most appropriate for use at night, although research is needed to substantiate this assertion.

Typically, nurses appear to use a combination of indices when making assessments, including verbal reports and behavioural and physiological signs. Jacox and Stewart (1973) and Oberst (1978) reported that in theoretical exercises, nurses inferred more pain from nonverbal than verbal communication. In clinical settings, Jacox (1979) found that nurses reported that physiological signs and behaviours were easier to interpret than verbal reports in pain assessment. Similarly, Saxey (1986) found that 69% of nurses in her sample reported that they used nonverbal methods such as facial expression and bodily movement as being the criteria most indicative of pain. Only 31% chose the patient's verbal report as the main assessment method.

Even though all the relevant pain research points to McCaffrey's conclusion that pain is what the patient says it is, it seems that nurses do not appear to act on verbal reports. If facial expression and body postures are generally used as the basis for the provision of pain control measures, problems of assessment are likely to be greater at night. Obviously in darkness nurses cannot observe patients easily, so that relying on what patients say becomes even more important.

Observing and talking to patients may be supplemented by more formalised methods of assessing pain. Various instruments have been devised, for example the McGill Pain Questionnaire (Melzack 1975) and the London Hospital pain observation chart (Raiman 1986). These instruments are quite complicated to use in clinical situations, requiring a considerable amount of effort from the patient either to complete them or provide the necessary information for the nurses to complete them. Simpler pain rating instruments are available, some of the more successful ones being verbal rating scales and visual analogue scales (Figures 6.1 and 6.2).

No pain at all

Discomfort

Moderate pain

Severe pain

Excruciating pain

Figure 6.1   Pain rating scale

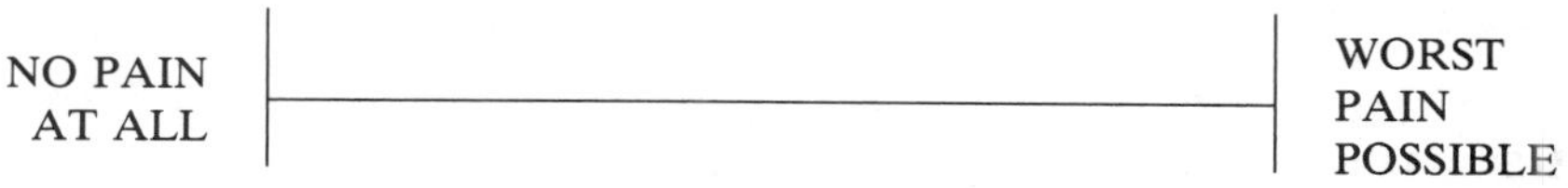

NO PAIN
AT ALL

WORST
PAIN
POSSIBLE

Figure 6.2   Pain Visual Analogue Scale

The line is 10cm long and patients are asked to place a mark across the line at a point indicating the intensity of their own pain. Pain is then scored by measuring how far along the line the mark was made. A similar scale can be used to assess pain relief, with the anchor words 'NONE' and 'COMPLETE' used instead. Such scales have been widely used with considerable success, although a few patients find it difficult to understand how to use them.

Simple pain assessment instruments have been used with considerable success in clinical situations. It is worth remembering, however, that even with the simplest of such instruments, considerable effort may be needed on the part of the patient to use them at night.

It is clear that there are many different ways of assessing pain. Since one of the aims of post-operative pain control is to avoid complications due to impaired mobility and breathing, a useful component of pain assessment might be to get the patient to move or cough so that any impairment can be observed.

It is not yet known how best pain and pain relief following surgery should be assessed at night, and work evaluating various methods in various combinations is needed.

Control of Post-operative Pain

There are various possible ways of controlling post-operative pain, many of which are complementary to standard pharmacological treatments. Not only are many of these therapeutic in their own right, but also they increase the individual's sense of having some control over the pain. When post-operative patients were asked whether they would consider using complementary therapies (Closs 1991), 56% said they would try relaxation, 49% the application of hot/cold pads, 46% distraction, 46% would try acupressure or massage, 32% hypnosis and 25% acupuncture. The four main methods patients had used spontaneously to manage their pain were physically supporting their wounds, deep breathing and relaxation, distraction and mobilisation. It appears that not only did a large proportion of patients show positive interest in using alternative pain control techniques, but also that many patients were already using some.

The remainder of this chapter discusses the merits of a range of complementary pain control techniques which may be of use to post-operative patients at night. These include patient-controlled analgesia (PCA) as well as cutaneous stimulation, hypnosis, acupuncture, transcutaneous electrical nerve stimulation, guided imagery, distraction and relaxation, with particular reference to the hospital setting. Many of these techniques could easily be learned by nurses and taught to patients.

Patient-controlled Analgesia

Since 'the only arbiter of pain is – or should be – the patient' (Rosen 1984) it makes a good deal of sense to allow patients to control their own pain relief regime. The concept of allowing post-operative patients to control the amount of opioid analgesic they receive is relatively new. Usually a pre-programmed infusion pump allows the patient to adjust the dose according to need, usually via intravenous and more rarely via epidural or extradural routes (Marlowe et al 1989). This method of administration avoids the peaks and troughs in serum levels of opioids produced by intramuscular administrations. Thus, effective analgesia is obtained because of the maintenance of a therapeutic level of narcotics in the blood. Tamsen and others (1982) reported of PCA that 'patients seem to self-administer narcotic analgesics in a consistent way . . . not in excess of usually recommended doses'. Contrary to expectations, the problem of respiratory depression has been minimal when using PCA. This method is particularly helpful at night, providing continuous analgesia while patients are asleep. If they wake because of pain, most systems allow them to give themselves a top-up dose which takes effect virtually immediately.

Kleiman et al (1987) found that nurses promoting the use of PCA suggested that 'the feeling of control that PCA provides may enhance patients' pain relief'. This was corroborated by Clark and others (1989) who observed that 'patients' anxiety and perceived intensity of pain may therefore be reduced because they are in control of their own pain relief'.

Virtually all research to date in this field suggests that the benefits of PCA to post-operative patients could be enormous. The major impediment to widespread introduction of PCA appears to be the belief that the cost of infusion equipment is prohibitive, currently about £2,000 each. This belief was challenged by Hecker and Albert (1988) who compared two different types of PCA pump and conventional analgesic therapy for efficacy and cost. They concluded that 'PCA provides superior pain management at minimal additional cost'. Although this method is cost-effective, finding the resources for the initial purchase of such equipment is likely to delay the widespread introduction of PCA.

Cutaneous Stimulation

Stimulation of the skin in order to reduce pain has been practised for centuries. The application of heat and cold and massage have produced various types and duration of pain relief (see McCaffery 1983). For the patient in pain at night, the various kinds of cutaneous stimulation provide a useful supplementary strategy.

According to Margo McCaffery (1990), the method of selecting an effective site for any cutaneous stimulation is one of 'trial and error combined with openmindedness'. There are various locations relative to the painful area which may provide successful analgesia. Usually (though not always) the best site is directly over or around the pain (Gammon and Staff 1941). If this is not successful, sites proximal (between pain and the brain) or distal (between pain and the periphery) may be more effective. McCaffery suggests that if these sites fail, trying an area contralateral (on the opposite side of the body) to the pain or an acupuncture point, or if all else fails, any site distant to the pain might still be successful.

Research ('Cooling more effective' 1982) has shown that local applications of cold to the knees of 100 patients suffering from rheumatoid arthritis and keen pain produced greater relief than heat. Interestingly however, patients tended to prefer heat since it produced less initial discomfort. It seems that alternate applications of heat and cold produced greater analgesic effect than either heat or cold alone. Even intermittent heat has proved effective in controlling severe pain. Allowing patients to develop their own timing for such applications is liable to produce optimum pain relief from this method. Intervals between applications may vary from 5 seconds to 20 minutes. This could be achieved by providing patients with two hot water bottles or even disposable rubber gloves filled with hot or iced water. This method would allow patients a greater sense of control over their pain. If being used at night (or with confused or frail patients), care should be taken that hot water bottles are not so hot as to burn the patient who may fall asleep during use.

Massage is another form of cutaneous stimulation which is claimed to produce beneficial therapeutic effects (Sims 1986, White 1988). While there is little rigorously conducted research to demonstrate these, numerous anecdotal sources suggest that massage can aid relaxation, decrease stress, decrease pain, distract from pain and improve sleep, among other benefits.

The type of cutaneous stimulation which has been demonstrated by research to produce beneficial therapeutic effects is the application of heat and cold. While other techniques such as massage could be used on a rather hit-and-miss basis, application of heat and cold shows considerable promise as a method of pain reduction available to patients.

Hypnosis

Hypnosis uses the power of suggestion to control pain, although how it achieves this is poorly understood. Hypnosis appears to produce a trancelike state where the subject's attention is focused on one thing only, usually the hypnotist. The subject experiences an altered state of consciousness, accompanied by a relaxed feeling. Once in this state different kinds of suggestion may be used to relieve pain (Hilgard and Hilgard 1986). The hypnotist may suggest that the painful area of the body is becoming numb, the numbness gradually increasing until the pain disappears. Alternatively, the idea of dissociation may be used, where the hypnotist separates the patient from his pain, perhaps by suggesting that the affected part is floating away from the patient's body, then returning without any pain.

Throughout this kind of procedure, the subject is not actually under the control of the hypnotist, although different people have the ability to be hypnotised to different 'depths'. It appears that about 30% of the population are able to attain a state of deep hypnosis, 30% a moderate level and 30% can reach a light, drowsy state. Mersky (1983, p 30) concludes from both clinical reports and personal experience that hypnotism is not 'worth using in anyone with pain of physical origin'.

Training is required in appropriate hypnotic techniques before nurses or patients attempt to use them. Although hypnosis does not immediately appear to be suitable for hospital patients, self-hypnosis might be a useful way to induce pain control or sleep for this particular group, and would be a useful area for some further research.

Acupuncture and Acupressure

Acupuncture is an ancient art and has been a traditional part of Chinese medicine for several thousand years. Traditionally, long, extremely fine needles are inserted into specific acupuncture points with the aim of harmonising the two life forces, yin and yang. Once the needle (which has a rounded end so that it pushes tissues apart rather than cuts them) has been inserted, the practitioner may twist, vibrate or heat the needle, or an electric current may be passed through it.

Much of the research which has examined the effectiveness of acupuncture in producing analgesia has concentrated on headache and back pain; very little has studied post-operative pain. Sung and others (1977) examined the effect of acupuncture on patients following wisdom tooth extraction. They found that acupuncture given with drug placebo gave significantly greater pain relief than sham acupuncture with a drug placebo.

Training is essential in order to practise acupuncture competently, so it is not a realistic option for most nurses. Acupressure, however, may be a method which could more easily be used in the clinical field. Hare (1988) suggested that 'acupuncture massage is particularly well suited for nurses, since the delivery of nursing care requires a high degree of touch sensitivity'. Acupressure is a technique whereby acupuncture points are stimulated by pressing or rubbing, producing similar effects to acupuncture itself. Shiatsu is a Japanese form of acupressure, and reflexology is yet another version. Of the effect of shiatsu on pain management and stress reduction, it has been suggested that it is 'a powerful tool when pain medication, sedation and tranquillisers must be avoided or reduced' (Hare 1988). Thus more evaluative work on the use of acupressure could produce valuable information for its effectiveness in reducing pain and stress and therefore enhancing sleep in post-operative patients.

Transcutaneous Electrical Nerve Stimulation (TENS)

This technique involves using a battery-powered generator to send mild electrical currents through the skin via adhesive electrodes. TENS may be used by patients with either chronic or acute pain, but is considered most effective where there is skin tenderness associated with nerve damage or disease (see Melzack and Wall 1988). Like PCA, it may produce a 'background' level of analgesia throughout the night, making sleep more likely.

Following surgery, electrodes may be placed on either side of the incision, though considerable expertise is required for the positioning to be effective. Either pre-operatively, or post-operatively when patients are feeling well enough, they may be taught how to regulate the electrical impulses so that they have some control over their pain.

The use of TENS for post-operative pain has produced conflicting findings. Hargreaves and Lander (1989) found that TENS significantly lowered pain levels during post-operative dressing changes. Gilbert et al (1986) found TENS ineffective for patients following inguinal herniorrhaphy, as did Stubbing and Jellicoe (1988) with thoracotomy patients. The latter group, however, had a significant reduction in nausea and vomiting. More research is needed before it is known whether or not TENS is an effective method in the treatment of pain following various types of surgery.

Guided Imagery

This technique may be described as purposeful or therapeutic use of mental images (McCaffery 1983). Such images may be purely visual, or may include all the senses. For example, imagining being on a beach includes not only the sight of the waves and sand, but also the sound and smell of the sea and the feeling of warm sun on the skin. Guided imagery is usually preceded by a relaxation exercise which then leads on to process imagery (for example the tide going out and taking the pain with it) and finally end-result imagery (such as lying pain-free on a peaceful empty beach with the sea out of sight).

More recently, research has shown an imagery technique known as sensory transformation had a significant effect on pain. Guided imagery was used to transform laboratory induced pain into a pleasant feeling (Geden et al 1984) with significant success. In 1987, Susan Vines studied the effect of guided imagery on the experience of unpleasant physical symptoms such as dental pain during root canal therapy, as well as arthritic and back pain. At least half of the sample of 62 subjects managed to alter their sensations, 10% achieved a reduction in blood pressure, while another 10% reported feeling more 'in control'.

As well as improving pain control, guided imagery has been shown to reduce emotional distress, nausea and physiological arousal (Burish and Lyles

1981) all of which are likely to disturb sleep, particularly in post-operative patients.

Distraction

This differs from guided imagery in that distraction depends on external stimuli while guided imagery depends purely on mental images. To quote Margo McCaffery, 'Distraction is a kind of sensory shielding, a protecting of one's self from the pain sensation by focusing on and increasing the clarity of sensations unrelated to pain' (1983). The patient's attention is focused on stimuli other than pain, tending to increase the ability to tolerate pain or to decrease its intensity. These effects are achieved by preventing pain from being the centre of the sufferer's attention. Simple devices such as listening to music or the radio, watching television, reading, or simply watching the goings on of a busy hospital ward can be used with considerable success. Nurses will be familiar with the phenomenon of a patient in pain perking up when visitors arrive, becoming apparently more cheerful until the visitors leave, when they revert back to an appearance of being in pain. Frequently these patients are not believed when they complain of pain, but it is likely that they were using distraction (in the form of visitors) to alleviate pain which returned as soon as the distraction ceased.

Patients should be encouraged to use any suitable kind of distraction, including reading, watching television, talking to nurses or one another, or simply observing what is going on around them. While this is possible during the day, it becomes more difficult at night when there is far less going on for patients to concentrate on.

Relaxation

This is perhaps the most important part of many of the techniques used to promote sleep and reduce pain. Titlebaum (1988) reviewed the literature on relaxation and concluded that it should be considered as a sense of control, promote sleep and reduce pain or the perception of pain.

Stresses including pain and anxiety cause an increase to sympathetic and motor nervous activity. These may produce an increase in pulse rate, respiratory rate, blood pressure and adrenalin secretion. In turn, these may produce feelings of irritability and tension, which disturb sleep, and may produce pain such as tension headaches. This may take place either directly, or indirectly by facilitating the activity of neurons that project pain signals to the brain. Much useful research in this area has been completed by Herbert Benson and his colleagues, who reviewed Eastern and Western religious and lay practices which led to the relaxation response. They found four common elements: a quiet environment, a mental device, a passive attitude and a comfortable position. They propose that the 'relaxation response' is the basis of all meditative practices, and causes specific physiological adjustments. Oxygen consumption is decreased, less carbon dioxide is eliminated, respiration rate and blood pressure are lowered (Benson et al 1977). Although they refined the technique in order to reduce stress, they acknowledge that it may help people to fall asleep. 'Some have even given up sleeping pills as a result' (Benson 1985).

The research which has attempted to evaluate the effect of relaxation on post-operative pain is difficult to evaluate, since different techniques have been used, with and without information-giving and not always considering the varying coping styles of patients. Wells (1982) studied cholecystectomy patients who had used relaxation as a method of post-operative pain management. She found that pain sensation was not reduced, but less distress was reported. Flaherty and Fitzpatrick (1978) used relaxation to aid the first post-operative attempt at getting out of bed following herniorrhaphy, haemorrhoidectomy or cholecystectomy. They found that it produced a significant reduction in the amount of analgesics required, incisional pain and body distress, and decreased respiratory rate. Miller (1987) used a deep breathing relaxation technique with a small sample of 15 post-operative patients with considerable success. She found a significant decrease in blood pressure, heart and respiratory rates and pain perception. Levin et al (1987) assessed the effectiveness of two relaxation techniques and found that rhythmic breathing had no significant effect on pain.

Overall, however, relaxation appears to have considerable potential for use with post-operative patients. Though further research could begin to pinpoint the optimum way to use the technique for this group, it appears that simple relaxation exercises could improve sleep and reduce pain for some patients.

Summary

Sleep and pain control are of considerable importance to the post-operative patient and there is great scope for the improvement of nursing assessment and treatment of pain at night. In particular, assessment skills need to be well-developed if nurses are to identify patients' problems quickly and accurately. Then nurses need the appropriate knowledge to help alleviate these problems. Perhaps in-service education from people who are experienced in some of the techniques discussed would be a useful way of supplementing nurses' knowledge and skills.

The alternative methods of pain control discussed in this chapter should be considered for use in addition to, not instead of standard pharmacological management. The methods which currently appear to hold the greatest potential for controlling post-operative pain at night appear to be PCA, cutaneous stimulation, acupressure, guided imagery and relaxation. Much more research into the efficacy of these techniques is required before more specific recommendations can be made.

Some patients may well benefit from trying some of these options regardless. While not all the pain control methods will work with every patient, some patience and persistence may pay off. A technique such as relaxation may not work the first time it is used, but may become progressively more effective with practice. If one strategy alone does not produce the desired effect, combinations of techniques may be successful.

There is considerable scope for innovation and imagination in the field of post-operative pain relief. The implementation and evaluation of some of these methods should allow nurses to increase their skills in these fundamental areas of night-time nursing care.

References

Akerstedt T and Froberg J E (1979) Sleep and stressor exposure in relation to circadian rhythms in catecholamine secretion. *Biological Psychology*, **8**, 869–880.

Bach S, Noreng M F and Tjellden N U (1988) Phantom limb pains in amputees during the first 12 months following limb amputation, after preoperative lumbar blockade. *Pain*, **33**, 3, 279–301.

Benson H (1985) The relaxation response. In Monat A and Lazarus R S (eds) *Stress and Coping. An Anthology*. Columbia University Press, 2nd edn.

Benson H, Koch J B, Crassweller K D and Greenwood M M (1977) Historical and clinical considerations of the relaxation response. *American Scientist*, **65**, 441–445.

Bing H I (1936) Viscerocutaneous and cutaneovisceral thoracic reflexes. *Acta Medica Scandinavica*, **89**, 57.

Bonica J J (1990) Post-operative pain. In Bonica J J (ed) *The Management of Pain* Volume 1. 2nd edition, Lea and Febiger: Philadelphia and London.

Bonica J J and Benedetti C (1980) Post-operative pain. In Condon R E and DeCosse J J (eds) *Surgical Care: A physiologic approach to clinical management* Lea and Febiger: Philadelphia, 394–414.

Burish T and Lyles J (1981) Effectiveness of relaxation training in reducing adverse reactions to cancer chemotherapy. *Journal of Behavioral Medicine*, **4**, 1, 65–79.

Burns J W, Hodsman N B A, McLintock T T C, Gillies G W A, Kenney G N C and McArdle C S (1989) The influence of patient characteristics on the requirements for post-operative analgesia. *Anaesthesia*, **44**, 2–6.

Carli G, Montesano A, Rapezzi S and Paluffi G (1987) Differential effects of persistent nociceptive stimulation on sleep stages. *Behavioural Brain Research*, **26**, 2–3, 89–98.

Clark E, Hodsman N and Kenny G (1989) Short report; improved postoperative recovery with patient-controlled analgesia. *Nursing Times*, **85**, 9, 54–55.

Clausen O P F, Thorud E, Bjerkness R and Elgjo K (1979) Circadian rhythms in mouse epidermal basal cell proliferation. Variations in compartment size, flux and phase duration. *Cell Tissue Kinetics*, **12**, 319–337.

Closs S J (1988) *A nursing study of sleep on surgical wards*. Nursing Research Unit Report, Department of Nursing Studies, University of Edinburgh.

Closs S J (1990) An exploratory analysis of nurses' provision of postoperative analgesic drugs. *Journal of Advanced Nursing*, **15**, 42–49.

Closs S J (1991) *A nursing study of night-time pain, analgesic provision and sleep following surgery*. Nursing Research Unit Report, Department of Nursing Studies, University of Edinburgh.

Cooling More Effective (1982) *Aches and Pains*, **3**, 37.

Craig K D, Prkachin K M (1983) Nonverbal measures of pain. In Melzack R (ed). *Pain Measurement and Assessment*. New York: Raven Press.

Donovan M, Dillon P and McGuire L (1987) Incidence and characteristics of pain in a sample of medical-surgical inpatients. *Pain*, **30**, 69–78.

Fielding J W, Fagg S L, Jones B G, Ellis D, Hockey M S, Minawa A, Brookes V S, Craven J L, Mason M C, Timothy A, Waterhouse J A H and Wrigley P F M (1983) An interim report of a prospective randomised controlled study of adjuvant chemotherapy in operable gastric cancer: British stomach cancer group. *World Journal of Surgery*, **7**, 390–399.

Fisher L B (1968) The diurnal mitotic rhythm in the human epidermis. *British Journal of Dermatology*, **80**, 75–80.

Flaherty G G and Fitzpatrick J J (1978) Relaxation technique to increase comfort level of postoperative patients: a preliminary study. *Nursing Research*, **27**, 352–355.

Gammon G D and Staff I (1941) Studies on the relief of pain by counter-irritation. *Journal of Clinical Investigation*, **20**, 13–20.

Geden E, Beck N, Hauge G and Pohlman S (1984) Self-report and psychological effects of five pain coping strategies. *Nursing Research*, **33**, 5, 260–265.

Gilbert J M, Gledhill T, Law N and George C (1986) *British Journal of Surgery*, **73**, 749–751.

Gobel H and Cordes P (1990) Circadian variation of pain sensitivity in pericranial musculature. *Headache*, **30**, 7, 418–422.

Hare M (1988) Shiatsu acupressure in nursing practice. *Holistic Nurse Practitioner*, **2**, 3, 68–74.

Hargreaves A and Lander J (1989) Use of transcutaneous electrical nerve stimulation for postoperative pain. *Nursing Research*, **38**, 3, 159–161.

Hecker B R and Albert L (1988) Patient-controlled analgesia: a randomized, prospective comparison between two commercially available PCA pumps and conventional analgesic therapy for postoperative pain. *Pain*, **35**, 115–120.

Hilgard E R and Hilgard J (1986) *Hypnosis in the Relief of Pain*, 2nd edn. Los Altos, Cal: William Kaufmann.

Horne J A (1983) Human sleep and tissue restitution: some qualifications and doubts. *Clinical Science*, **65**, 569–578.

Jacox A K (1979) Assessing pain. *American Journal of Nursing*, **74**, 491–495.

Jacox A K and Stewart M (1973) *Psychosocial Contingencies of the Pain Experience*. Iowa City: University of Iowa College of Nursing.

Katz R (1977) Informed consent: is it bad medicine? *Western Journal of Medicine*, **126**, 426–428.

Kleiman R L, Lipman A G, Hare B D and Macdonald S D (1987) PCA vs. regular IM injections for severe postop pain. *American Journal of Nursing*, Nov, 1491–1492.

Levin R F, Malloy G B and Hyman R B (1987) Nursing management of post-operative pain: use of relaxation techniques with female cholecystectomy patients. *Journal of Advanced Nursing*, **12**, 463–472.

McCaffery M (1983) *Nursing the Patient in Pain*. London: Harper and Row.

McCaffery M (1990) Nursing approaches to nonpharmacological pain control. *International Journal of Nursing Studies*, **27**, 1, 1–5.

Marks R M and Sachar E J (1973) Undertreatment of medical inpatients with narcotic analgesics. *Annals of Internal Medicine*, **78**, 2, 173–181.

Marlowe S, Engstrom R and White P F (1989) Epidural patient-controlled analgesia (PCA): an alternative to continous epidural infusions. *Pain*, **37**, 97–101.

Melzack R (1975) The McGill pain questionnaire: major properties and scoring methods. *Pain*, **1**, 277–299.

Melzack R and Wall P (1988) *The Challenge of Pain*, 2nd edn. London: Penguin Books.

Mersky H (1983) The psychological treatment of pain. In M Swerdlow (ed.) *Relief of Intractable Pain*, Amsterdam: Elsevier.

Miller K (1987) Deep breathing relaxation – a pain management technique. *AORN Journal*, **45**, 2, 484–488.

Nimmo W S and Duthie D J R (1987) Pain relief after surgery. *Anaesthesia and Intensive Care*, **15**, 68–71.

Oberst M T (1978) Nurses' inferences of suffering: The effects of nurse-patients similarity and verbalisations of distress. In Nelson M J (ed.) *Clinical Perspectives in Nursing Research*, 38–60. New York: Teachers College Press.

Pollman L and Hildebrandt G (1987) Circadian profiles and circaseptan periodicity in the frequency of administration of analgesic drugs after oral surgery. *Functional Neurology*, **2**, 2, 231–237.

Raiman J (1986) Towards understanding pain and planning for relief. *Nursing (London)*, **11**, 411–423.

Rigas B, Torosis J, McDougall C J, Vener K J and Spiro H M (1990) The circadian rhythm of biliary colic. *Journal of Clinical Gastroenterology*, **12**, 4, 409–414.

Rosen M (1984) Patient controlled analgesia. *British Medical Journal*, **289**, 640–641.

Saxey S (1986) The nurses' response to post-operative pain. *Nursing*, **10**, 377–381.

Seers C J (1987) *Pain, Anxiety and Recovery in Patients Undergoing Surgery*. PhD thesis, University of London.

Shaver J, Giblin E, Heitkemper M and Paulsen V (1989) Sleep and its restorative function. *Communicating Nursing Research*, **22**, 80.

Sims S (1986) Occasional paper: slow stroke back massage for cancer patients. *Nursing Times*, **82**, 47, 47–50.

Sriwatanakul K, Weis O F, Alloza J L, Kelvie W, Weintraub M and Lasagna L (1983) Analysis of narcotic analgesic usage in the treatment of postoperative pain. *Journal of the American Medical Association*, **250**, 7, 926–929.

Stubbing J F and Jellicoe J A (1988) Transcutaneous electrical nerve stimulation after thoracotomy. *Anaesthesia*, **43**, 296–298.

Sung Y F, Kutner M H, Cerine F C and Frederickson E L (1977) Comparison of the effects of acupuncture and codeine on post-operative dental pain. *Anesthesia and Analgesia; Current Researches*, **56**, 473–478.

Tamsen A, Hartvig P, Fagerlund C, Dahlstrom B and Bondesson U (1982) Patient-controlled analgesic therapy. *Acta Anaesthesiological Scandinavica*, **Suppl 74**, 157–160.

Titlebaum H M (1988) Relaxation. *Holistic Nurse Practitioner*, **2**, 3, 17–25.

Valk I M and Van Den Bosch J S G (1978) Intra daily variation of the human ulnar length and short term growth – a longitudinal study in eleven boys. *Growth*, **52**, 107–111.

Weitzman E D, Zimmerman J C, Czeisler C A and Ronda J (1983) Cortisol secretion is inhibited during sleep in normal man. *Journal of Clinical Endocrinology and Metabolism*, **56**, 352–358.

Wells N (1982) The effect of relaxation on postoperative muscle tension and pain. *Nursing Research*, 31, 236–238.

White J A (1988) Touching with intent: therapeutic massage. *Holistic Nurse Practitioner*, **2**, 3, 63–67.

Woolf C J (1983) Evidence for a central component of post-injury pain hypersensitivity. *Nature*, **306**, 686–688.

Chapter 7
Nurse-patient Relationships at Night: A Psychosocial Perspective
Louise de Raeve

'At night time it would be an enormous comfort to the patient if the nurse sat with him, even if no words were spoken'

(Holgate 1988)

This seemingly simple request forms the starting point of a chapter which will explore some of the interpersonal dynamics that may underlie nurse-patient relationships and since the focus of this book is on night nursing, as much illustrative material as possible will be taken from night nursing literature. It is my belief that interpersonal skills can only be taught through an interpersonal process of learning, so this chapter will deliberately not provide a 'how to do it' guide to therapeutic interventions. What will be addressed is an exploration of some aspects of 'emotional care' (Nichols 1984), followed by a consideration of the phenomenon of 'regression' in illness and a brief introduction to the concept of 'transference'. The idea that illnesses often have profound and highly individual meanings for patients will then be explored in conjunction with the significance of this phenomenon for nurse-patient relationships, particularly with regard to information giving. This chapter will have a bias towards general nursing but will hopefully still be of interest to nurses working in the fields of psychiatry and mental handicap.

Emotional Care

To return to Mr Holgate's statement, most nurses would probably feel that provided time allowed, such a request could be easily met. However this was not Mr Holgate's experience. This raises the following questions: what was the nature of the need being expressed, how should such needs be evaluated in relation to physical needs and how able are nurses to meet them?

Roy Holgate's need seems to have been profound. His article is a description of his hospital experience at night following a coronary by-pass operation. He states 'nights in hospital came to fill me with horror' and 'Although my body was healing, my fears at night were increasing and I delayed going to bed as much as possible'. Speculation about the possible causes of such a reaction might lead us to think about the meaning of the night for somebody who has had major surgery at the 'heart' of their being: the possible equation of darkness with death, the parallels of loss of consciousness in sleep with fears of death and the anaesthetic experience and so forth. He describes going through a period of uncertainty about his body and of feeling that 'minor matters became magnified at night'.

Dodds' (1980) research revealed that 'many patients seem to feel isolated and vulnerable during the night, and unpleasant incidents were therefore magnified and remembered'. This is not surprising information; 'lying awake worrying' and 'getting things out of proportion' at night are common experiences for all of us. If one adds to this the patient's experience of being far from home, in an unfamiliar and relatively impersonal environment, of being in physical discomfort if not actual pain and of facing tremendous uncertainty it is perhaps surprising that people manage to sleep at all in hospital.

Mr Holgate's need, it would seem, was considerable. What might have prevented it from being understood? Firstly of course, it might not have been expressed clearly. It is sometimes hard to find the right words to express emotional needs and to believe in oneself that such needs are legitimate. One may hope that the other person will somehow 'tune in' or 'pick up' the cues and 'know' what is required without anything having to be specifically stated. This puts the onus for understanding squarely in the lap of the nurse which is perhaps both a little unrealistic and a little unfair. Relatively few nurses will have experienced a major operation themselves and even fewer will have had heart surgery. We need to be given the chance to learn from the patients within our care about what it is they require. However there may be several factors which restrict our receptively to requests for 'emotional care' (Nichols 1984).

Nurses working at night may themselves feel lonely and isolated (Pryde 1987). There may be feelings of resentment at having had to refuse an invitation out with friends, at having had to rush the family meal or leave a husband comfortably watching television and there may be some very mixed feelings about enabling others to sleep while having to try to keep awake oneself. This could perhaps explain why nurses do not always seem to be attentive in trying to minimise noise at night (Dodds 1980, Royal Commission of the NHS 1978).

Apart from specific responses to the experience of night duty, our individual receptivity to requests for emotional care will vary according to our personal mood, our belief in our abilities to meet such needs and our sense of priorities in nursing care. Dodds (1980) quotes the rather distressing example of a patient crying about the death that evening of a patient in the next bed and calling to the nurse for comfort: 'The nurse told her firmly to "pack it in" and "go to sleep" '. This is a clear example of 'blocking': a verbal response which effectively prevents all further communication on the subject (Macleod-Clark 1981). Without knowing more of the context it is impossible to understand what went wrong, but it seems reasonable to conclude that for whatever reason, the patient's request presented the nurse with something she could not cope with and had to fend off. In so doing the inability to cope was made to be totally the patient's problem and remained disowned by the nurse. What this scenario underlines is that if we cannot emotionally cope with something, no matter what the reason and we cannot acknowledge this limitation to ourselves and others, then our capacity to care will be diminished and our propensity for cruelty increased, when patients raise issues which touch upon these areas.

We all have moods, we all have vulnerabilities and we all have crises in our personal lives to deal with. It is not that the ability to give good emotional care requires us to be superhuman, rather it requires us to be able to acknowledge how human we are. The person who comes on duty knowing they are in a mood and knowing what sort of a mood it is, is in a very different position from the person who is in a mood but has given no thought to the matter. For one thing, one may be able to let others know that one is not functioning at one's best. Colleagues and patients are then relieved of the anxiety of wondering if they've done or said something 'wrong' and are mentally prepared to perhaps make some allowances.

It has been suggested that apart from personal moods, belief in our ability to meet requests for emotional care would affect our receptivity to such requests. As nurses we are great 'doers'. It is perhaps simultaneously our strength and our weakness. We are prepared to do for others what many people would not contemplate doing, but on the other hand the need to 'do' can interfere with the capacity to just 'be'. Being with someone and doing nothing may involve us in powerful feelings of helplessness. We can't bring a dead person back to life, we can't always change the course of an illness, we may feel impotent in the face of deep emotional pain. One of the problems is that because we feel so helpless and impotent, we tend to assume that this is our failing, that somehow we should know what to do or say to make things better. Faced with our limitations in this respect, we then tend to retreat back into the world of physical activity where our competence seems less in question and the patient will perhaps be referred to the perceived experts: the social worker or nurse counsellor, etc.

While such referrals may be totally appropriate, they may sometimes be based on a misapprehension about what such skills entail. It isn't that trained counsellors know 'what to do' any more than the average nurse. The feelings of vulnerability and helplessness are part of the reality of the situation and cannot be 'taught away'. What counsellors learn to do is to tolerate such feelings, so that they can reflect upon them and continue to be with the person rather than having to take flight. While full training in counselling skills is a lengthy process (and not to be confused with brief introductory courses) all nurses who are prepared to reflect upon themselves would be able to extend their capacity for giving emotional care provided they could be supported by individual or group supervision. A starting point could be peer supervision to shift handovers. As Nichols (1984) says of emotional care:

> The most fundamental requirement though, has to be that someone in an executive position (doctor, ward sister etc) does regularly ask, concerning each person on the ward, 'who is handling this person's psychological care and how is it going?'

The question that remains to be asked is 'is this psychological/emotional care important' and if so, 'why'? At the beginning of this chapter it was suggested that most of us would have felt that Mr Holgate's request could be met 'provided time allowed'. That time 'might not allow' suggests that other things could take precedence and we have just explored how as individuals we may give priority to the world of doing for, rather than being with, patients, as a defensive response to our own sense of inadequacy. However, this pattern of behaviour may extend beyond individuals and become part of the institutional or organisational system which in turn exerts its own pressure on individuals to conform. It could be said that the collective perception of emotional care as being of secondary importance to that of physical care, is a collective defensive strategy (Menzies 1970).

Wilson-Barnett (1978a) comments that 'It is surely very short-sighted to provide psychological comfort only when nurses "have time" as this may be of equal value to many physical care procedures'. It was Querido (1959) who demonstrated in a research study of 1,630 patients that the presence of distress (defined as 'social and/or psychic tensions too heavy for the patient to bear') created a discrepancy between the predicted favourable clinical outcome and the actual clinical outcome. The latter was reduced by approximately 50%. Querido (1959) states:

> 'Even if the phenomenon of 'distress' is regarded merely as a plodding and worrying attitude to life or as a psychological peculiarity of the patient, it is plain that such a mental attitude on the part of the patient reduces the efficiency of the hospital by almost half.'

If we fail to address this problem as nurses, it could be said that we are merely doing half a job. Roy Holgate's experience bears testimony: 'having asked for help had the nurses sat with me for a minute or two – even without speaking – my panic and distress would have subsided'.

Making gentle enquiries as to the nature of a patient's feelings and allowing time and space to listen to the reply may not only help prevent the negative effects of emotional distress on recovery, it may also facilitate recovery. Nichols (1984) states 'they [emotional reactions] often signify important psychological processes of adaptive preparation and adaptive change. The processes can usually be aided by direct and frequent expression of the feelings involved to another person. . .'

To be helpful we sometimes need to do very little apart from listen attentively and make quiet the voice within us that thinks we should be able to do more. We also have to be prepared to accept the 'No thank you' of patients who may not wish to use us in this way. The capacity to listen attentively can however be enhanced by an understanding of some of the dynamics of nurse-patient interactions. Therefore it is now pertinent to explore the three previously mentioned phenomena of regression, transference and the emotional meaning of illness to the individual patient.

Regression

Regression has been defined as a 'return to earlier ways of coping with psychological stresses' (Blumenfield and Thompson 1985) and by Weddell (1955a) as follows: 'In situations of stress and anxiety, some of the ideas, feelings and ways of behaving at a younger age or stage of development may be returned to – illness may be such a situation'. The potty trained toddler who reverts to bed wetting at night on the birth of a sibling is displaying regressive behaviour. One important feature of regression is that it is not with the individual's conscious control. The toddler has not decided to behave in this way, which is why punishment as a response would be quite inappropriate.

As McGhie (1979) observes: 'Regression is usually a transient reaction, the individual returning to a more mature way of acting when the stressful situation is alleviated'. Alleviation does not of course mean that the external situation necessarily changes, the sibling is going to be forever present after all, but what may change is the way in which the event is perceived. As the little child regains confidence in the belief that there is still a place for her in her parents' affections, that she is still loved and essentially good despite her anger, the stress and anxiety subside and the symptom of bed wetting normally disappears.

Regression can be described in both positive and negative terms. McGhie (1979) sees it as 'The avoidance of present difficulties by a reversion to an earlier, less mature, way of adjustment to the situation'. An everyday example would be staying at home with a headache rather than 'facing the music' at work, and we can probably all think of examples of patients who seemed reluctant to embark on the rehabilitation process, despite the amelioration of their physical condition: the passivity of dependence being seen as in some way preferable to the struggle for independence.

Temporary regression may, however, have a very positive function. It may allow the individual time to 'take stock' and re-assess priorities. It may permit an experience of being cared for that is needed. Peplau (1988) suggests that 'needs unmet in the past are often revived or intensified during illness'. If this is so then one could perhaps see illness as offering a 'second chance' to be given the care that one was deprived of during some earlier developmental phase. The regressive aspects of physical illness, the relinquishing of self care and responsibility to others, could also be seen as freeing emotional and physical energy, thereby permitting a degree of self-centredness and inner orientation to enable the individual to concentrate on 'getting better'.

The question arises as to whether or not physical illness is a particular manifestation of a more general regressed state or simply a condition which brings about regressive behaviour. Either way however, other people's responses to physical illness certainly invite regression. This can be seen in the withdrawal from the everyday world that illness legitimises. This may be followed by a dependence on others for meals and physical care. Others may become interested in one's inputs and outputs in a way reminiscent of early infancy and so on. What are the implications of regression in illness for nursing?

As a general nurse one responds without much thought or question to the more routine tasks of bedmaking, serving of meals, coaxing to eat, emptying of bedpans etc. However there are situations where the way forward is not always clear. The person who seems to have a vested interest in perpetuating their dependency beyond the time that their physical condition would warrant requires very careful nursing. Is this just a period of temporary resistance: the two steps forward and one back of most patterns of progress, or is it a sign of something more entrenched? The nursing assessment would require information about the meaning of the patient's resistance and this might take time to discover. Lydia Hall (1969) gives a very good illustration of this kind of difficulty. She describes the situation of a patient admitted for rehabilitation who refused to participate in a programme of progression from bed to wheel-chair, preferring to stay in bed. That the patient eventually decided to by-pass the wheelchair stage entirely and to walk instead, suggests that he received impressive physical and emotional nursing care. It is our loss that Lydia Hall's article does not record all the significant nursing interventions that led to this outcome.

It may not always be constructive to meet regressed demands for care and dependency but it is essential to respond to such requests and demands with understanding. As nurses we also have to acknowledge that there is a tend-ency to give patients very mixed messages. On the one hand for example, we expect people to pursue their post-operative physiotherapy with enthusi-asm but on the other hand we implicitly state that we don't believe any patient is capable of making the tea, let alone serving it to others: that is the province of the domestic staff.

Firmness as a nursing response may sometimes be appropriate but this is not to be confused with control, bullying or retaliation. A lot has been said so far about the importance of meeting emotional care needs but one may need to try to distinguish between need and greed and between realistic and unrealistic expectations. Some people may feel they deserve instant service. This tends to produce an understandable irritation in nurses who resent being perceived to be at someone's 'beck and call'. The problem is what to do with the irritation. If it is unacknowledged, the chances are that the nurse will say she is coming back in a minute and then forget to do so, leaving the patient with a mounting sense of frustration. As was stated at the beginning of this chapter, there are no recipes or prescriptions for how best to respond, it would depend upon the context and the personalities of the people involved. However, what one can say is that patients need to know the effect they have on the nurse and nurses need to make clear what their limitations are and to try to understand why he feels as he does. Without this, there is no way either party can proceed to work more realisitically together.

This raises the question of whether or not one should express one's anger or irritation directly to patients. There is no rule that says that nurses should not and to do so may provide both patient and nurse with food for thought and underline the honesty of the relationship. To do so, regret it and apologise may also be perceived by patients as honest and may enable patients to feel that they are not the carriers of all the weakness while the nurses have all the strengths. However, one needs to be cautious: patients are vulnerable in their illness. The angry response of the night nurse previously described would have merely served to enhance the patient's isolation and misery. There is a great difference between situations where anger is used to totally reject a person and an angry interchange that occurs within the context of a more accepting relationship where there is the chance for further engagement and resolution. The source of the anger is also important to consider. If it is one's own bad mood then it should not be patients who have to help one cope with it.

Where nurses feel that they are frequently angry or irritated with a patient it is important to discuss this with colleagues: not just to establish whether or not others feel similarly but to take the thinking further in an effort to understand why. People who successfully provoke anger in others are usually angry themselves and anger may be a mask for many other feelings, including fear, helplessness and worthlessness (Franks 1985). If the underlying feeling or feelings can be understood, the anger may subside.

A prickly, angry, complaining response is one quite common way that regressive behaviour in illness is manifested. Other manifestations might include passive submission or the jokey person who is the 'life and soul of the party'. What determines these different responses to hospitalisation and illness? The first factor would be the patient's personality and their particular 'coping strategy' (Johnson and Lauver 1989): that is their characteristic way of coping with stress, the foundations of which will have been determined in early childhood. The second factor likely to determine the particular pattern of regression is the meaning the illness and its symptoms have for the patient. The experience of previous hospital admissions and illnesses would also have an influence (Blumenfield and Thompson 1985).

All patterns of response and adaptation have their strengths and weaknesses and respective implications for nursing. The person who copes with hospitalisation by being the life and soul of the party tends to be popular with nurses (Stockwell 1972). However while joviality may imply underlying adjustment it may sometimes mask underlying anxiety. If, as nurses, we are too 'seduced' by our perception of such a person as being fun to be with and able to cope, we may miss an important dimension. It could be for example that such a person has a considerable fear of the repercussions of alienating nursing staff and consequently has to work very hard at keeping things agreeable.

In returning to examine these three illustrations of regressive behaviour; the passive submissive person, the prickly person and the jokey person, we can now perhaps see how the nurse is being perceived in three different ways. The passive submissive person has, seemingly at least, relinquished much personal responsibility and handed it over in the belief that doctors and nurses know what to do best. The prickly person is in a fight with us over control and the jolly person wants to be our friend. It is suggested that none of these perspectives accurately reflects the nurse-patient relationship as it in fact is: adult to adult. Each view or way of relating involves a slight distortion: another element or dimension is present. This dimension has been termed the transference.

Transference

It was the psychoanalyst Freud who first identified this phenomenon and it refers to a situation whereby relationships in the present are invested with past meaning that comes from our early childhood relationships with significant others (usually parents and siblings) (Tschudin 1987). Because of the nature of our work as nurses and the position that patients find themselves in, in relation to us, the transference we are most likely to receive is a maternal (and sometimes paternal) one. The sex of the nurse influences which it is, although it does not depend exclusively upon this. In other words, patients may be partly relating to us as they did in childhood to their mothers or fathers. This phenomenon is not within the individual's control and the person is not usually conscious of it. If the individual does become aware that they are behaving in this way, the power of the transference is likely to diminish or disappear. For most of us, transference is only ever part of the picture. With the exception of those people who are psychotically ill or demented, no one is actually going to believe we really are their father or mother.

If we return to our three illustrations and now look at them from the perspective of the possible nature of the maternal transference they could be re-described like this: for the passive submissive patient the nurse has become the idealised, omniscient and omnipotent mother, for the prickly patient the transference is a negative one towards a failing, threatening controlling mother figure and with the jolly person the transference could again be of a threatening mother figure resulting in a response which makes it safer to turn nurses into friends and thus de-professionalise and disempower them. These are gross generalisations. To understand what transference phenomena may be operating in a particular situation, one needs to have detailed information, gathered over time, so that one can begin to see what patterns of interaction emerge.

The concept of transference can enable us to make sense of our experiences when we find ourselves in the middle of confusing and powerful forces in relationships with patients and where we feel we are not being seen quite as we actually are. It can help us to regain a certain objectivity. When patients fall in love with their nurses it is likely to be because the phenomenon of transference is operating. In other words it is the patient's love for his or her mother that is being partially projected on to the nurse. Understanding possible transference phenomena may be helpful to nurses but because of the unconscious nature of the process, it is not normally advisable for such hunches to be shared with patients, unless of course the patient gives the lead.

Transferences can of course work both ways and we as nurses may also see patients as 'mothers', 'fathers', 'brothers', 'sons' and 'daughters' etc. It is important to try to identify this in ourselves. A strong positive or negative reaction to a patient we hardly know could be an indication that this process is operating and would suggest the need for some inner reflection and perhaps supervision. Without such inner detective work, we are in danger of simply acting out an inner scenario in the external world, with the patient as an unwitting accomplice. This process can interfere with our capacity to give effective nursing care as we may be unable to see the patient and his needs as he truly is.

The Meaning of Illness

A further factor, apart from transference but related to it, that may influence the nature of a person's regression in illness is the meaning that the person attributes to his illness and its symptoms. If a person believes that their illness is a punishment from God for misdemeanours known or unknown, then it isn't hard to imagine that the illness is likely to be experienced as a deeply threatening attack on that person's psychological sense of integrity. The patient's response to medical and nursing staff will inevitably be coloured by this picture. Nurses are likely to be seen as accusers or punishers rather than allies in the transition from illness to health.

This is a rather extreme example but we can probably all recall enounters with patients where it became clear that their perception of what was happening to their bodies had little to do with the realities of human physiology. An example in the author's experience is of a man who in the terminal stages of rectal cancer had developed pronounced ascites. He seemed deeply relieved to be informed that this was a colourless, odourless liquid that had nothing to do with urine or faeces.The power of these imaginings is made worse in the presence of uncertainty and the absence of real information but it would be a mistake to assume that factual information necessarily mitigates against these ideas. This is because the source of what one imagines is happening is less to do with the rational intellectual self and much more to do with the inner world of feelings, of the unconscious and of memories and imaginings from childhood (Weddell 1955b).

How might we as nurses 'tune into' the meanings that our patients may be giving to their illness? People are likely to hide these beliefs, feeling perhaps that they have no place in the clear cut, clinical world of hospital life; that they are 'silly' and will be laughed at or disbelieved and so forth. Sometimes it may also be hard to find the words to describe them. It will not be until a relationship of trust has been established that we could hope to be entrusted with such deeply personal information and of course we need to create the physical and emotional space to receive such communications. Nevertheless there are ways in which we could begin. How much time for instance do we give when admitting a patient to really allow that person to describe their illness in their own terms and how much time do we spend thinking about this communication afterwards?

Language has symbolic content and there may be many layers of meaning behind an apparent statement of fact. To take a deceptively simple example, 'I have a headache' is not likely to be just a statement about a physical pain in my head. It may well refer to the pain in my mind as well. We accept this mind-body connection in an everyday way when we commonly acknowledge that one gets headaches when emotionally stressed but the wisdom of this lay understanding seems to get lost in hospital life with the dominance of the biomedical model (Engel 1977). If we are prepared to listen for them, patients may give us clues as to their underlying beliefs about their illness, in their everyday communications.

The meaning that a patient may be giving to his illness has important implications for the giving of information. Much research has been done into exploring the importance of information giving and into what style or type of information is most useful to patients (Hayward 1975, Boore 1980, Wilson-Barnett 1978a and b, Johnson and Lauver 1989, and Ridgeway and Mathews 1982). However, presumably because of the necessity for standardising responses in the interest of measurability, none of these research studies addresses the idea that perhaps the most helpful information would be that which tries to meet precisely what it is the individual seems to want to know. Perhaps some people are very relieved by descriptions of likely sensations whereas for others this is less relevant. It seems obvious that the kind of information one seeks will be related to the kind of anxieties one has and the kind of anxieties one has will be related to the meaning one is giving to the experience. Trying to establish what the patient's specific worries are should perhaps be the precursor of any nursing attempts at information giving.

Working with Colleagues

So far, the whole of this chapter has deliberately focused on nurse-patient relationships. However before concluding, it seems important to look briefly at the context within which these relationships take place; the multi-disciplinary team. Mention has already been made of the necessity for sharing with colleagues one's experiences of nurse-patient interactions, for purposes of supervision and support. However a stronger point needs to be made about the importance of working together.

Nievaard's (1987) research showed that: 'The more problem-ridden the relations were with doctors and management, the more negative the nurses' attitudes were to their patients'. A positive attitude of nurses to patients was found to 'coincide with a reduction in hospitalisation problems like isolation and displacement'. One might therefore legitimately surmise that a negative attitude to patients will be likely to compound these same problems, which might in turn have implications for the patients' rate and degree of recovery (Querido 1959).

As nurses therefore who are concerned to maximise the therapeutic potential and minimise the non-therapeutic impact of our relationships with patients, it becomes clear that we have a duty to work at developing and sustaining good collegial relationships. This requires a preparedness to confront and try to work through interpersonal difficulties with colleagues. The implications for the relationship of day and night nurses should also be evident. As Joan Kemp (1985) remarks: 'It is unfortunate when information relating to a patient's abilities and psychological state fails to cross the day-night divide so that the significance of the 24-hour processes is ignored'. Both day and night nurses need to be truly interested in, and respectful of, each others' 'stories'. The picture that best describes the patient's reality is likely to be the one that is a synthesis of all the various views, not the picture that the most dominant voice or team describes.

To conclude, this chapter has attempted to explore a few of the common underlying dynamics of nurse-patient interactions. Much more remains to be said and much more remains to be discovered. No matter what our starting point, we can all develop our capacity to give better emotional care provided we are prepared to look at ourselves and have the chance to receive some degree of external support or supervision.

References

Blumenfield M and Thompson T (1985) The psychological reactions to physical illness. In Simons R (ed.) *Understanding Human Behaviour in Health and Illness* (3rd edn). London: Williams and Wilkins.

Boore J (1980) Information – a prescription. *Nursing Mirror*, Dec 11 1980.

Dodds E J (1980) *Slept Well? A study of ward activity and nurse-patient interaction at night*. Unpublished MSc dissertation.

Engel G (1977) The need for a new medical model: a challenge for Biomedicine. *Science*, **196**, 129–136.

Franks R D (1985) The difficult patient. In Simons R (ed.) *Understanding Human Behaviour In Health and Illness* (3rd edn). London: Williams and Wilkins.

Hall L (1969) The Loeb Centre for Nursing and Rehabilitation, Montefiore Hospital-and Medical Center, Bronx, New York. *International Journal of Nursing Studies*, **6**, 81–97.

Hayward J (1975) *Information – a prescription against pain*. RCN.

Johnson J E and Lauver D R (1989) Alternative explanations of coping with stressful experiences associated with physical illness. *Advances in Nursing Science* Jan, **11**, 2, 39–52.

Kemp J (1985) It's different at night. *British Journal of Geriatric Nursing*, **5**, 5, 20–22.

McGhie A (1979) *Psychology as Applied to Nursing* (7th edn). Edinburgh: Churchill Livingstone.

Macleod Clark J (1981) Communication in nursing. *Nursing Times* Jan 1, **77**.

Menzies I (1970) *The Functioning of Social Systems as a Defense Against Anxiety*. London: Tavistock Publications.

NHS Royal Commission (1978) Patients' attitudes to the hospital service. *NHS Royal Commission Research Paper no 5*.

Nichols K A (1984) *Psychological Care in Physical Illness*. London: Croom Helm.

Nievaard, A C (1987) Communication climate and patient care: causes and effects of nurses' attitudes to patients. *Soc. Sci. Med*, **24**, 9, 777–784.

Peplau H (1988) *Interpersonal Relations in Nursing*. Basingstoke: Macmillan Education Ltd.

Pryde N A (1987) Night nursing for trainees: living up to the image. *International Nursing Review*, **34**, 3, 80–83.

Querido A (1959) Forecast and follow-up. An investigation into the clinical, social and mental factors determining the results of hospital treatment. *British Journal of Prev. Soc. Med.*, **14**, 33–49.

Stockwell F (1972) *The Unpopular Patient*. RCN.

Tschudin V (1987) *Counselling Skills for Nurses*. London: Bailliere Tindall.

Weddell D (1955a) Psychology applied to nursing. *Nursing Times*, Jan 28.

Weddell D (1955b) Psychology applied to nursing. *Nursing Times*, Feb 11.

Wilson-Barnett J (1978a) In hospital: patients' feelings and opinions I and II. I *Nursing Times*, March 16, 29–32. II *Nursing Times*, March 23, 33–34.

Wilson-Barnett J (1978b) Patients' emotional response to barium X-rays. *Journal of Advanced Nursing*, **3**, 37–46.

Some Useful Addresses

The British Association For Counselling
1 Regent Place, Rugby CV21 2PJ
Tel: 0788 578328

Psycho-Dynamic Understanding In Nursing
Organising Tutor: Mrs Anna Dartington
The Tavistock Clinic
120 Belsize Lane, London NW3 5BA
Tel: 071 435 7111

Course in Counselling In Health Care Settings
Birkbeck College
University of London, 26 Russell Square, London WC1
Tel: 071 636 8000 ext. 3826

Chapter 8
Nurses as Nightworkers

Peter Totterdell, Lawrence Smith and
Simon Folkard

Having to work at night can cause a range of problems for an individual and
for his employer. The individual may experience disruptions to her or his
sleep, health and social life and this may lead to increased absenteeism and
reduced performance and safety at work. However, in some professions such
as nursing there is an unavoidable requirement to provide a service at night
and it is therefore important that nurses and nursing managers should understand the specific problems of working at night so as to minimise its disruptive
effects.

Circadian Rhythms

Many of the problems of nightwork result from the fact that we have evolved
as a diurnal species. That is, our bodies are geared up to be awake and active
during the day and asleep at night. Consequently, most of our social activities
and customs have also developed to accommodate this pattern.

The Body Clock

Many of our physical and even mental processes have been shown to vary in
a predictable fashion over the course of 24 hours (e.g. Folkard 1983). This
cyclic behaviour has been termed a circadian rhythm; ciradian meaning 'about
a day'. These rhythms are set by our 'body clock'. It is not known whether
there is more than one master clock but experiments have isolated a particular
area of the brain's hypothalamus as playing a role in controlling at least some
of these rhythms (Stephan and Zucker 1972).

Studies in which humans have been isolated from all time cues for long
periods of time have shown that the natural period (the time a rhythm takes
to reach the same point in its cycle) of the clock is in fact nearer to 25 than
24 hours (e.g. Wever 1979). Some rhythms, such as the sleep-wake cycle, are
less strongly coupled to the clock and by 'shortening' or 'lengthening' the day
using artificial time cues the rhythms can be made to 'break out' from the
clock to show their own natural periods (e.g. Folkard et al 1983). However,

in everyday life we use cues from the environment, such as the light-dark cycle and social cues such as meal times to entrain the rhythms to cycle once every 24 hours or thereabouts. Normally this keeps us 'in tune' with our environment, and probably once conferred us with an evolutionary advantage. Unfortunately this system is not adapted for nightwork.

Adjustment

The problem with nightwork is that individuals have to try to sleep when their rhythms are preparing them for wakefulness and activity, and have to work when their rhythms are at their lowest ebb and their resistance to sleep is at a minimum. Over a series of night duties the circadian system begins to adjust but different rhythms adjust at different rates causing disturbance of the circadian system. Adjustment can take several weeks and it is possible that for many individuals the system may never fully adjust (Knauth and Ilmarinen 1975).

The general feelings of malaise that can result from this disturbance are similar to those experienced in jet lag. However, with jet lag the situation is considerably better because all the environmental cues in the new time zone help the circadian system to adjust. With nightwork the environmental cues encourage the circadian system to remain on a diurnal schedule.

Working permanently on nights may be the best solution to the problem because it gives the body a chance to adapt. However, this will only work if the individual remains on a nocturnal routine (active at night, asleep during the day) on their days off becaue the circadian system adjusts more quickly back to a diurnal routine (Knauth et al 1981). It is quite clear that, because of social pressures, most nightworkers in fact revert to a diurnal routine on their days off. The alternative is to minimise disruption to the circadian system, rather than encouraging adjustment, by utilising rotating shift systems in which the individual employee only works 2 or 3 night shifts consecutively and then works another type of shift.

Sleep

Nightworkers often have problems sleeping and this may be at the root of many of the other physical problems associated with nightwork. About 60–70 per cent of shift workers complain of sleep disruption (Rutenfranz et al 1985). The average length of daytime sleep of a group of 157 permanent female nightworkers was found to be 6 hours and 6 minutes (Gersten et al 1986) and for a group of 29 full-time permanent nurses was 6 hours and 10 minutes (Verhaegen et al 1987). Curtailed sleep is often attributed to social and environmental factors such as increased noise and disturbances during daytime sleep. Undoubtedly these factors play a part but the body clock is also responsible.

Research on shiftworkers and in laboratory studies has shown that there is a strong relationship between the time of day at which sleep begins and the subsequent duration of the sleep (e.g. Zulley et al 1981). The ease with which people can fall asleep also depends on the time of day (Lavie 1986). The results show that there is only a four hour period between 22:00 and 02:00 during which people are likely to be able both to fall asleep easily and subsequently to sleep for seven or more hours.

From other research it would seem that people often start to have problems such as fatigue, stress and irritability when their sleep falls below about seven hours on a number of successive days. This means that if you are working nights, and therefore trying to sleep outside of 22:00 to 02:00 hours, then your body clock won't allow you to sleep as much as you need. In a study of 1,505 female hospital workers, Estryn-Behar et al (1990) found that by comparison with the morning shift, women on the night shift were at a higher risk of sleep impairment and fatigue, and scored worse on a measure of mental health.

However, most of this discussion has been based on average figures for sleep; actual figures may vary from one individual to the next. They also vary according to age. Older people typically have more sleep problems and may therefore find it more difficult to adapt to nightwork (e.g. Akerstedt and Torsvall 1980). Then again, older nightworkers are sometimes the ones that have found ways of adapting to nightwork and have managed to stick with it.

Performance and Safety

The evidence in the shiftwork literature suggests that both impaired performance and safety tend to be associated with night work and this impairment is due to the combined effects of disrupted circadian rhythms and partial sleep deprivation (Folkard and Monk 1979). Performance speed is reduced while error and the potential for more serious accidents are increased (Folkard 1987). However, it is worth noting that a lot depends on the nature of the task being performed and work conditions. For example, performance might be susceptible on either a monotonous monitoring task, or when crucial decisions are being made under a heavy workload and distracting conditions. Many performance capabilities are naturally at their lowest ebb during the early hours of the morning. When this is combined with low levels of alertness, a lessened ability to resist sleep, work fatigue, and the effects of a possible sleep debt built up over successive night shifts, then efficient task performance may be compromised.

In one study of over 400 night nurses, Folkard, Condon and Herbert (1984) reported the occurrence of a phenomenon known as 'night shift paralysis'. This condition is a form of sleep paralysis (Goode 1962) which occurs during the transition between wakefulness and sleep when falling asleep, and, more rarely, when waking up. It usually occurs in the early hours in night workers who are performing a sedentary task, but who are subsequently required to make some movement, perhaps to attend to a monitor alarm, or a distressed patient. Night shift paralysis is characterised by a temporary inability to make gross movements, even though the individual is aware of what it is they have to do. This state may last for several minutes, and although it is a relatively rare phenomenon its incidence has implications for both performance and safety. Night shift paralysis was reported to have been experienced by 12 per cent of the night nurses in the above study. One associated factor appeared to be reports of feeling sleepier than usual.

Social and Family Life

The full extent to which unusual work hours affect the social and family lives of shiftworkers is difficult to determine because there is such large variation in both individual charactersitics and preferences, as well as in the nature of shift systems, type of work, length of shifts and so on (e.g. Wedderburn 1975). Impoverished family and social lives are amongst the most common complaints reported by shiftworkers. The disruptive effects are a result of the work and non-work periods of shiftworkers being 'out of step' with their normal social environment. Broadly speaking shiftwork can affect the social pattern of a person's life in terms of:

1. The membership of organisations and taking part in regular institutionalised activities. Shiftworkers are less likely to be active members of an organisation such as a parent-teacher association, political party, civic group, etc, or to hold office within them once they have joined (Walker 1985). Regular participation in organised sports and other recreational activities may be limited because they are usually geared towards the evening time and weekends. There are also severe limitations upon opportunities for further training or education. All of which may have a cost attached in terms of personal fulfilment and well-being.
2. The quality and quantity of contact with family and friends. To some extent the evidence here is more equivocal, however, research has suggested a 'two-step' effect upon family life. Firstly, there is the conflict between the positioning of work and rest periods, and the time usually devoted to valued family activity. In addition, nightworkers may spend considerable time 'recovering' on rest days following a block of night shifts. They may also be more irritable and less able to interact well with other family members. Secondly, these conflicts may have a cumulative interfering effect upon family and marital relationships (Mott et al 1965). The nightworker may not be able to provide as much companionship, emotional support and protection, nor fulfil the more initmate, sexual role with a partner. If both partners are shiftworkers (especially on different shift schedules) then contact time may be considerably diminished. However, some shiftworking couples with children choose such an arrangement so that there is always someone available to provide child care. Shiftworkers may be particularly disadvantaged when it comes to attending important social or family functions such as anniversaries, weddings, etc, or are not free on public holidays when a lot of social activity occurs. Walker (1985) noted that such conflicts with family roles may interact with mental health to affect self-esteem and emotional well-being. On the social side, shiftworkers may have fewer friends than

dayworkers and those that they do have tend to be other shiftworkers. Moreover, their irregular work hours may mean that they are excluded from many of the activities that their friends arrange, further increasing a sense of isolation.

3. The opportunity to fulfil domestic commitments. Shiftworkers may be at more of an advantage than dayworkers with respect to taking children to and from school, going shopping, visiting the bank or post office, making use of welfare facilities, undertaking home improvements, etc, and may be more flexible in terms of visiting relatives. Many women shiftworkers will tend to be disadvantaged, because they are, more often than not, responsible for the daily upkeep of a household, the provision of meals, etc. This 'double burden' may be a source of considerable strain, especially when personal welfare takes second place to looking after the family and domestic work (Gadbois 1980).

4. Participation in solitary, or near solitary activities. Once again, those shiftworkers who enjoy solitary hobbies and activities such as gardening, fishing, walking, reading and so on, may benefit from having more time to devote to these pastimes than dayworkers. However, as stated above, those who prefer group activities, e.g. going to the cinema or having a meal with friends, playing a team sport, may suffer from impoverished social contact.

Health Risks

Most of the health problems associated with nightwork which we have referred to so far have been ones which manifest themselves relatively quickly, such as sleep disruption, fatigue, stress and irritability. In the long term, however, the strain of nightwork can either increase susceptibility to or cause more serious health problems. One of the difficulties in determining long-term effects, however, is that current nightworkers are often a self-selected 'survivor population'; and the greatest problems are often found in the group of workers who have had to transfer on to daywork.

Gastrointestinal Disorders

Shiftworkers experience increased incidence of gastrointestinal disturbance, including: loss of appetite, constipation, heartburn, stomach pains and flatulence. And more seriously they are also more likely to develop peptic ulcers (e.g. Costa et al 1981).

There are a number of possible contributory factors. Altered sleep patterns produce changes in the central nervous system and endocrine mechanisms. The internal disturbance which results may produce a state similar to that found in stress induced ulcer disease (Vener et al 1989). Meal times are known to be important synchronisers for some physiological circadian rhythms (Reinberg 1974), and therefore changes to meal times may also contribute to the internal disturbance. The composition as well as the timing of meals is also commonly altered during nightwork and this may also have an effect. Nightworkers typically increase their consumption of carbohydrates in the form of snacks (Cervinka et al 1984).

Cardiovascular Disease

Some recent Swedish research (Knuttson 1989) has shown that there is an association between shiftwork and Coronary Heart Disease (CHD). The research has shown that the greater the number of years of exposure to shiftwork the greater the risk of heart disease, even when other possible factors such as increased levels of smoking are taken into account. So as well as increasing the risk indirectly, by causing changes in smoking habits for example, shiftwork also appears to have a more direct effect in increasing the risk of heart disease, probably via disturbed physiological mechanisms.

Mortality

So far there is very little evidence that shiftworkers die younger. In a study of over 8,000 male manual workers, carried out over a period of 13 years, Taylor and Pocock (1972) found that the death rate for day workers, shiftworkers and ex-shiftworkers was not statistically different from the national death rate. The rates for different causes of death were also similar amongst the different groups. However, in a comparison of four printing groups: rotary printers, plate makers, compositors and correctors, Teiger (1984) found that the rotary printers, who were the only group on permanent nights, died prematurely in larger numbers and earlier than the other groups both before and after retirement. The rotary printers also had more long-term sick leaves and had the highest percentage of early retirement through incapacity. The four groups had the same order of occupational risk but given that the groups did slightly different jobs, work environment rather than night work cannot be ruled out as the cause of overmortality in this case.

Psychiatric Disorders

A number of studies, but by no means all of them, have found that shiftworkers have a higher incidence of neurotic disorders such as anxiety and depression (e.g. Costa et al 1981).

Medical Checks

Given the evidence that nightwork is a risk factor for health problems, regular health checks before, during and after assignment to nightwork are recommended. Health measures for shiftworkers (e.g. Koller 1989) commonly suggest that individuals should be exempted from nightwork if they suffer any of the following (e.g. Koller 1989):

- gastrointestinal disorders such as gastric ulcers;
- diabetes, especially insulin-dependent, because of the need for proper food intake and timing of medication;

- epilepsy because sleep deficit may increase the chance of a seizure;
- chronic heart disease;
- severe nervous disorders because they can often be influenced by the sleep-wake cycle.

Practical Measures

There are a variety of different ways in which the problems of nightwork can be reduced. The stress and strain model of shiftwork (Colquhoun and Rutenfranz 1980) distinguishes between the external stress which comes from the shift system itself and the internal strain which develops in the individual as they attempt to cope with the shift system. The options, therefore, are to intervene both at the organisational level to reduce the stressful effects of the shift system, perhaps by adopting a new shift system, and at the individual level to reduce the strain that the individual experiences, perhaps by training them to adopt useful behavioural strategies.

Shift Systems

Nurses work a variety of shift systems. Night shifts may either be part of a rotating shift system, in which the nurse works morning, afternoon and night shifts, or they may be part of a permanent shift system in which the nurse works only night shifts (either for a block of weeks or always) and a different nursing workforce covers the daytime hours.

There is often a greater flexibility in terms of swapping and requesting particular shifts than in other professions. This makes it essential that those responsible for arranging the duty rota should know something of the rules of good practice. Unless permanent nights are in operation, the number of successive nights should be minimised so as to reduce disruption of the circadian system and prevent a build up of sleep deficit (Akerstedt 1985).

In a rotating system the shifts should 'delay'; that is they should start later than the previous one, such as Morning to Afternoon to Night, rather than 'advance' such as Morning to Night to Afternoon (Czeisler et al 1982). There are two reasons for this. Firstly, a delaying system encourages a later sleep start time which is more in line with the 25 hour body clock. Secondly, a delaying system avoids 'quick returns' where there are only a few hours between the end of one duty and the start of the next. A 'quick return' does not allow sufficient recovery time.

The timing and duration of shifts are also important. The morning shift should not start too early because social pressures and the body clock combine to stop individuals sleeping earlier than normal the night before (Folkard et al 1990). This will also probably be better from the patient's viewpoint (patients have body clocks too!) because it means that they won't be woken so early.

However, it would probably be better to start the night shift later rather than increase its duration because long shifts can result in fatigue. Some organisations are now using 12 hour shifts because by condensing the working week it gives the employee longer breaks and there is some evidence that this reduces sickness (Lees and Laundry 1989). A number of studies have compared nurses on 8 and 12 hour shifts. In a study of 10 inpatient wards who changed from 8 hour to 12 hour shifts, Todd et al (1989) found that the quality of care decreased on 12 hour shifts. In another comparison, Johnston et al (1989) found that the nurses on 12 hour shifts tended to be less alert and worked significantly faster but less accurately on mental performance tests. And finally, although Fields and Loveridge (1988) found no difference in fatigue or critical thinking between nurses on 8 and 12 hour shifts, the results did indicate that the 12 hour night nurses were more drowsy.

Naps

Taking a nap before or, where allowed during, a night shift may have beneficial effects. In a study involving nurses, Harma et al (1989) found that the 56 per cent of nurses who took a nap before the first night shift had better sleep quality and were more alert during the shift particularly towards the end of the shift. The length of the nap did not seem important. Smith and Wilson (1990) found that nurses who took a nap in the middle of a shift had problems immediately following the nap but felt better and performed better on mental performance tests towards the end of the shift.

Fitness

There is evidence that improving fitness may also improve adaptation to nightwork. Harma et al (1986) found that a group of nurses who undertook a fitness training programme for four months were more alert and performed better on memory tests than a control group, especially on night shift.

Diet

Given the gastrointestinal problems experienced by nightworkers, it has been suggested that the situation can be improved by paying closer attention to dietary factors. In particular, it is recommended that meal times should be kept as regular as possible. High carbohydrate and high fat meals should be avoided during the night shift.

Medication

Sleeping pills or hypnotics are not recommended for nightworkers. Any benefit obtained will only be short term and using such drugs on a regular basis may lead to problems on withdrawal. What is needed is a drug which can reset the circadian system to accommodate the new routine. So far melatonin has looked the most promising drug. It has helped in alleviating some of the problems of jet-lag (Arendt 1986) but more recent work suggests that it may also have detrimental effects on performance.

Alcohol should also be avoided as a means of getting to sleep because it can reduce the quality of sleep. Similarly, large amounts of caffeine should be avoided as a means of keeping awake.

Coping

Individuals develop their own strategies for coping with nightwork; some are more successful than others. Folkard et al (1978) found that the circadian rhythms of full time night nurses showed greater adjustment than those of part time night nurses. Having ruled out a number of possible reasons for the difference, the authors concluded that the most plausible explanation was that the full-timers were making more of a commitment in life-style to accommodate working at night. In another study of night nurses, Adams et al (1989) found that those nurses who adapted to nightwork better than their personality measures would predict tended to be very disciplined in their use of time and to 'sacrifice' their social activities.

Overall, little research has been done on the ways in which shiftworkers reduce, or cope with, the disruptive effects of their work schedules. Thus, the extent to which the *causes* of shiftwork problems and the *problems* themselves are engaged and managed, accepted or avoided is relatively unknown in shiftwork populations. Although speculative at present, it seems reasonable to suggest that for the 60 per cent who appear to endure shiftwork, for whatever reasons, personal resourcefulness and coping skills may play a significant role in how these individuals manage themselves and the situation, and importantly, how it affects their well-being. Research is now under way, by the Shiftwork Research team at the Social and Applied Psychology Unit, Sheffield, which will examine how shiftworkers cope, and what situational and personal factors influence this process.

Suitability for Nightwork?

Much of our discussion so far has centred on groups of nightworkers, but in fact it would be misleading to suggest that individuals respond uniformly to nightwork. It has been estimated that up to 30 per cent of shiftworkers leave shiftwork within the first few years of shiftwork due to health problems. But then again up to 10 per cent of shiftworkers are said to positively enjoy working shifts. In this section we try to identify those types of individuals likely to suffer least from nightwork.

It is well established that circadian rhythms differ from one individual to another along a number of dimensions, including: when the rhythm peaks, its size, its stability and its rate of adjustment. A number of questionnaires have been developed to distinguish between personality types based on these dimensions and attempts have been made, with some success, to relate these personality types to shiftwork tolerance.

Individuals who feel at their best earlier in the day are referred to as morning types, whilst others who feel at their best later in the day are referred to as evening types. Morning types tend to go to bed earlier and their circadian rhythms normally peak earlier in the day than evening types. A number of questionnaires have been devised which distinguish between morning and evening types (e.g. Horne and Ostberg 1976). A slightly modified version of this questionnaire is reproduced below so that you can assess whether you are a morning or an evening type. Simply decide which of the alternative answers to each question fits you best, and then check the scoring key at the end of this chapter. Add up your scores on each question to derive your total morningness score.

According to Horne and Ostberg's (1976) classification, if you score 70 or more (the maximum is 86) you are a Definite Morning Type, between 59 and 69 you are Moderate Morning Type, between 42 and 58 you are Neither Type, between 31 and 41 you are a Moderate Evening Type, and below 30 (the minimum is 16) you are a Definite Evening Type. It should be noted that only about 10 per cent of people fall into the definite Morning (5 per cent) or Evening (5 per cent) type categories, and that most people (about 60 per cent) fall into the Neither type category.

A number of studies have examined the relationship between morningness scores and people's ability to cope with shiftwork. Perhaps not surprisingly, Morning Types generally experience more problems coping with the night shift, but fewer problems coping with an early morning shift. Conversely, Evening Types have fewer problems on the night shift, but more on an early morning shift. However, there is little evidence that morningness scores relate to people's ability to cope with a rotating shift system, presumably because the advantages and disadvantages on different shifts cancel one another out on such a system. Thus any advantage or disadvantage to being a definite Morning or Evening Type is probably confined to shiftworkers who work permanent night or early morning shifts.

Categorising people according to their ability to sleep at different times of day (flexibility) and their ability to overcome drowsiness (vigorousness) has proved rather more successful in predicting people's ability to cope with a rotating shift system (Costa et al 1989). A Circadian Type Questionnaire has been developed to measure these dimensions of individual difference (Folkard et al 1979) and is currently being validated in a number of studies. If successful, it should allow the identification of those people best (or least) able to cope with a rotating shift system before they start working on it, and might thus be used for selection or guidance purposes.

Women Nightworkers

In this section, we look at those issues which particularly affect women working at night.

Women have a range of reasons for working at night including (from Wedderburn 1989):

- work only available at night;
- free time in the day;
- higher earnings;
- more time for family and house work;

The Morningness Questionnaire

1. Considering your own 'feeling best' rhythm, at what time would you get up if you were entirely free to plan your day?
   (a) before 06.30 (b) 06.30–07.44 (c) 07.45–09.44 (d) 09.45–11.00 (e) after 11.00

2. considering your own 'feeling best' rhythm, at what time would you go to bed if you were entirely free to plan your evening?
   (a) before 21.00 (b) 21.00–22.14 (c) 22.15–00.29 (d) 0.30–01.45 (e) after 01.45

3. If there is a specific time at which you have to get up in the morning, to what extent are you dependent on being woken up by an alarm clock?
   (a) not at all dependent (b) slightly dependent (c) fairly dependent (d) very dependent

4. Assuming adequate environmental conditions, how easy do you find it getting up in the mornings?
   (a) not at all easy (b) not very easy (c) fairly easy (d) very easy

5. How alert do you feel during the first half-hour after having woken in the morning?
   (a) not at all alert (b) slightly alert (c) fairly alert (d) very alert

6. How is your appetite during the first half-hour after having woken in the mornings?
   (a) very poor (b) fairly poor (c) fairly good (d) very good

7. During the first half-hour after having woken in the morning, how tired do you feel?
   (a) very tired (b) fairly tired (c) fairly refreshed (d) very refreshed

8. When you have no commitments the next day, at what time do you go to bed compared to your usual bedtime?
   (a) seldom or never late (b) less than one hour later (c) 1–2 hours later (d) more than two hours later

9. You have decided to engage in some physical exercise. A friend suggests that you do this one hour twice a week and the best time for him is between 7.00–8.00 a.m. Bearing in mind nothing else but your own 'feeling best' rhythm, how do you think you would perform?
   (a) would be on good form (b) would be on reasonable form (c) would find it difficult (d) would find it very difficult

10. At what time in the evening do you feel tired and as a result in need of sleep?
    (a) before 21.00 (b) 21.00–22.14 (c) 22.15–00.44 (d) 00.45–02.00 (e) after 02.00

11. You wish to be at your peak performance for a test which you know is going to be mentally exhausting and lasting for two hours. You are entirely free to plan your day and considering only your own 'feeling best' rhythm, which ONE of the four testing times would you choose?
    (a) 08.00–10.00 (b) 11.00–01.00 (c) 15.00–17.00 (d) 19.00–21.00

12. If you went to bed at 11.00 p.m. at what level of tiredness would you be?
    (a) not at all tired (b) a little tired (c) fairly tired (d) very tired

13. For some reason you have gone to bed several hours later than usual, but there is no need to get up at any particular time the next morning. Which ONE of the following events are you most likely to experience?
    (a) will wake up at usual time and will NOT fall asleep
    (b) will wake up at usual time and will doze thereafter
    (c) will wake up at usual time but will fall asleep again
    (d) will NOT wake up until later than usual

14. One night you have to remain awake between 04.00–06.00 in order to carry out a night-watch. You have no commitments the next day. Which ONE of the following alternatives will suit you best?
    (a) would NOT go to bed until watch was over
    (b) would take a nap before and sleep after
    (c) would take a good sleep before and nap after
    (d) would take ALL sleep before watch

15. You have to do two hours of hard physical work. You are entirely free to plan your day and considering only your own 'feeling best' rhythm, which ONE of the following times would you choose?
    (a) 08.00–10.00   (b) 11.00–01.00   (c) 15.00–17.00   (d) 19.00–21.00

16. You have decided to engage in hard physical exercise. A friend suggests that you do this for one hour twice a week and the best time for him is between 10.00–11.00 p.m. Bearing in mind nothing else but your own 'feeling best' rhythm, how well do you think you would perform?
    (a) would be on good form   (b) would be on reasonable form
    (c) would find it difficult   (d) would find it very difficult

17. Suppose that you can choose your own work hours. Assume that you worked a FIVE hour day (including breaks) and that your job was interesting and paid by results. At what time would you choose to START your five hours work?
    (a) 22.00–02.00   (b) 03.00–04.00   (c) 05.00–11.00   (d) 12.00–16.00
    (e) 17.00–21.00

18. At what time of day do you think you reach your 'feeling best' peak?
    (a) 05.00–07.00   (b) 08.00–09.00   (c) 10.00–16.00   (d) 17.00–21.00
    (e) 22.00–04.00

19. One hears about 'morning' and 'evening' types of people. Which ONE of these types do you consider yourself to be?
    (a) Definitely a 'morning' type
    (b) Rather more a 'morning type than an evening type'
    (c) Rather more an 'evening' than a 'morning' type
    (d) Definitely an 'evening' type

- more responsibility at work;
- greater freedom from supervisors;
- better atmosphere at work.

In a UK survey of shiftworkers (Robson and Wedderburn 1990), 79 per cent of women with children gave domestic circumstances as one of their reasons for working shifts, compared to 14 per cent of wives without children, and 13 per cent of married men. Of single women, 60 per cent worked shifts because it was part of the job, compared to 56 per cent of men and 36 per cent of married women.

Legislation

Until 1988 there was a legal prohibition on women working at night in the UK. However, certain sectors such as nursing were exempt from this prohibition and other exceptions were granted on a case by case basis, often on the grounds of economic expediency.

The prohibition of women working at night was enshrined in the International Labour Office's Convention No. 89, 1948, on Night Work (Women). In recent years, however, the legislation has been seen as discriminatory and running counter to directives on equal treatment of the sexes. The revised ILO proposal, yet to be approved, recommends that exemptions be granted by agreement between organisations representative of the employers and organisations representative of the workers. The prohibition on night work will, however, still apply during the 3 months before and 3 months after childbirth, unless the individual concerned makes a specific request to work and provided that the health of the woman or child will not be endangered. The prohibition will also apply to additional periods during and after pregnancy on production of a medical certificate. It is proposed that the income of the employee be protected during these periods.

However, there are some who argue that removing protective legislation is more likely to be in the interests of the employer than in the interest of equal opportunities (e.g. Coussins 1979) and that what is needed is better protective legislation covering both sexes. The European Social Charter may prove to be of relevance here in its directives on work time.

Gender Differences

Research has shown that shiftwork is a risk factor for the health and well-being of both male and female workers. But is there any evidence to suggest that women shiftworkers are at greater risk than their male counterparts or indeed that there are any additional considerations that need to be taken into account? In his review of the somewhat scanty research in this area Singer (1989) concluded that:

- where female and male shift workers are compared in survey type studies, women usually show greater satisfaction and better ability to cope;
- female/male comparisons on biological variables show no differences;
- from the research reviewed, no case can be made for differential legislation.

Based on a large-scale study of night nurses in France, Estryn-Behar et al (1990) found no sex related differences in health but found that women were twice as likely to be tired and irritable. However, women with children fared worse on these scales than either childless women or men with or without children. These differences can probably be attributed to the 'double burden' of domestic work rather than to some biological difference, and in particular to the fact that the women are likely to get less sleep as a result of their domestic work.

Gadbois (1980) showed quite clearly that for night nurses with family responsibilities, domestic duties take priority over sleep. He found that the daytime sleep of a group of unmarried nurses was on average 1 hour and 20 minutes longer than that of a group of nursing auxiliaries who were married with two children. The auxiliaries were more likely to go to bed later in order to get the children off to school and their sleep was more likely to be interrupted for the midday meal.

Menstrual Cycle

There has been very little research on the possible interaction between disturbances of the daily body rhythms caused by nightwork and the monthly rhythm of the menstrual cycle. An interaction between different shifts and the phase of the menstrual cycle on ratings of physical discomfort has, however, been found (Pokorski et al 1990). In a study of day and night workers employed as either nurses or telephone operators, Uehata and Sasakawa (1982) found higher rates of menstrual problems, such as irregular cycles and severe pains, among the night workers. A higher number of clinic visits for menstrual problems among night workers has also been recorded (Colligan et al 1979). However, not all studies find these effects.

Pregnancy

In his review of this topic, Costa (1990) shows that although the findings are not clear cut, quite a large proportion of studies have suggested that night work is probably a risk factor for pregnancy. Uehata and Sasakawa (1982) found higher rates of fertility problems, abortion and stillbirths amongst night workers. Some studies have indicated a higher risk of miscarriage (e.g. Axelsson et al 1984) but others have failed to confirm this finding (e.g. Axelsson et al 1989). A number of studies, but by no means all, have also found an association between night work and pre-term delivery (e.g. Axelsson et al 1989).

Social Considerations

The BEST report (Wedderburn 1989) on Women and Nightwork highlights some of the other problems that women face in working at night, including sexual harassment, danger in travelling to and from work, and fear at night.

One study found that in their sample, the number of women night workers reporting sexually harassing events was twice as high as during the daytime (Knauth and Schonfelder 1988). In a study involving health care services, De Lange (1983) found that the proportion of employees experiencing fear was higher amongst women, was much higher amongst women with respect to travel to work, and was higher on the night shift than the evening shift for both sexes but was much worse for women. Given these and some of the other issues raised in this section, there is a clear requirement for nursing management to address conditions of work for night nurses with respect to security, transport and child care.

Concluding Remarks

Nightwork, with its potential disruptive influence, will always be part of the nursing profession. Many nightworkers face problems, in terms of their physical and psychological well-being, by virtue of the fact that they are required to be out of step with both the natural rhythms of their bodies and their social environment. There is hope to be gained, however, in the knowledge that both the judicious choice of shift systems and the provision of personal coping information to nightworkers will help reduce the disruptive effects of working at night.

References

Adams J, Folkard S and Young M (1989) Coping strategies used by nurses on night duty. *Ergonomics*, **29**, 2, 185–196.

Akerstedt T (1985) Adjustment of physiological circadian rhythms and the sleep-wake cycle to shiftwork. In Folkard S and Monk T H (eds) *Hours of Work – Temporal Factors in Work Scheduling*. New York: Wiley.

Akerstedt, T and Torsvall L (1980) Age, sleep and adjustment to shiftwork. *5th Eur. Congr. Sleep Res.* Amsterdam, 190–195.

Arendt J, Aldhous M and Marks V (1986) Alleviation of jet lag by melatonin: preliminary results of a controlled double blind trial. *Br. Med. J.* **292**, 1170.

Axelsson G, Lutz C and Rylander R (1984) Exposure to solvents and outcome of pregnancy in university laboratory employees. *Br. J. Ind. Med.*, **41**, 305–312.

Axelsson G, Rylander R and Molin I (1989) Outcome of pregnancy in relation to rregular and inconvenient work schedules. *Br. J. Ind. Med.*, **46**, 393–398.

Cervinka R, Kundi M, Koller M and Haider M (1984) Shift related nutrition problems. In Wedderburn A and Smith P (eds) *Psychological Approaches To Night and Shift Work*. Edinburgh: Heriot-Watt University.

Colligan M J, Frockt I J and Tasto D L (1979) Frequency of sickness absence and worksite clinic visits among nurses as a function of shift. *Journ. Environ. Pathol. & Toxicol.*, **2**, 135–148.

Colquhoun W P and Rutenfranz J (eds) (1980) *Studies of Shiftwork*. London: Taylor and Francis.

Costa G (1990) *Shiftwork: Effects on Well Being & Health*. Unpublished manuscript. Institute of Occupational Medicine, University of Verona, Italy.

Costa G, Apostoli P, D'Andrea F and Gaffuri E (1981) Gastrointestinal and neurotic disorders in textile shift workers. In Reinberg A, Vieux N and Andlauer P (eds) *Night and Shift Work: Biological and Social Aspects*. Oxford: Pergamon.

Costa G, Lievore F, Casaletti G, Gaffuri E and Folkard S (1989) Circadian characteristics influencing interindividual differences in tolerance and adjustment to shiftwork. *Ergonomics*, **32**, 4, 373–385.

Coussins J (1979) *The Shift Work Swindle*. NCCL Rights for Women Unit.

Czeisler C A, Moore-Ede M C and Coleman R M (1982) Rotating shift work schedules that disrupt sleep are improved by applying circadian principles. *Science*, **217**, 460–463.

De Lange W (1983) *Working irregular hours in the health and care services*. Tilburg: Catholic High School [in Dutch].

Estryn-Behar M, Gadbois C, Peigne E, Masson A and Le Gall V (1990) Impact of nightshifts on male and female hospital staff. In Costa G, Cesana G, Kogi K and Wedderburn A (eds) *Shiftwork: Health, Sleep and Performance*, 89–95. Frankfurt Main: Peter Lang.

Estryn-Behar M, Kaminski M, Peigne E, Bonnet N, Vaichere E, Gozlan C, Azoulay S and Giorgi M (1990) Stress at work and mental health status among female hospital workers. *Brit. Journ. Ind. Med.*, **47**, 1, 20–28.

Fields W and Loveridge C (1988) Critical thinking and fatigue: how do nurses on 8 and 12 hour shifts compare? *Nursing Economics*, **6**, 4, 189–191.

Folkard S (1983) Diurnal variation. In Hockey G R J (ed.) *Stress and Fatigue in Human Performance*, 245–271. Chichester: Wiley.

Folkard S (1987) Circadian rhythms and hours of work. In Warr P B (ed.) *Psychology of Work*, (3rd edn). London: Penguin.

Folkard S and Monk T H (1979) Shiftwork and performance. *Human Factors*, **21**, 483–492.

Folkard S, Arendt J and Clark M (1990) Sleep, mood and performance on a 'weekly' rotating (7-7-7) shift system: some preliminary results. In Costa G, Cesana G, Kogi K and Wedderburn A (eds) *Shiftwork: Health, Sleep and Performance*, 484–490. Frankfurt Main: Peter Lang.

Folkard S, Condon R and Herbert M (1984) Night shift paralysis. *Experientia*, **40**, 510–512.

Folkard S, Monk T H and Lobban M C (1978) Short and long-term adjustment of circadian rhythms in 'permanent' night nurses. *Ergonomics*, **21**, 10, 785–801.

Folkard S, Monk T H and Lobban M C (1979) Towards a predictive test of adjustment to shift work. *Ergonomics*, **22**, 1, 79–91.

Folkard S, Wever R and Wildgruber C M (1983) Multi-oscillatory control of circadian rhythms in human performance. *Nature*, **305**, 223–226.

Gadbois C (1980) Women on night shift: interdependence of sleep and off-the-job activities. In Reinberg A, Vieux N and Andlauer P (eds) *Night and Shift Work Biological and Social Aspects*, 223–229. Paris: Pergamon Press.

Gersten A H, Duchon J C and Tepas D I (1986) Age and gender differences in night workers' sleep lengths. In Haider M, Koller M and Cervinka R (eds) *Night and Shiftwork: Longterm Effects and Their Prevention*, 475–477. Frankfurt Main: Verlag Peter Lang.

Goode G B (1962) Sleep paralysis. *Archives of Neurology*, **6**, 228–234.

Harma M J, Ilmarinen, I, Knauth P, Rutenfranz J and Hanninen O (1986) The effect of physical fitness intervention on adaptation to shiftwork. In Haider M, Koller M and Cervinka R (eds) *Night and Shiftwork: Longterm Effects and their Prevention*, 221–229. Frankfurt Main: Verlag Peter Lang.

Harma M, Knauth P and Ilmarinen J (1989) Daytime napping and its effects on alertness and short-term memory performance in shiftworkers. *Int. Arch. Occup. Environ. Health*, **61**, 341–345.

Horne J and Ostbert O (1976) A self assessment questionnaire to determine morningness-eveningness in human circadian rhythms. *International Journal of Chronobiology*, **4**, 97–110.

Johnston M, Pollard B, Manktelow A and Stavrou A (1989) *Stress and Information Processing in 8- and 12-hour nursing shifts*. Psychology Unit, Royal Free Hospital, London.

Knauth P, Emde E, Rutenfranz J et al. (1981) Re-entrainment of body temperature in field studies of shift work. *Int. Arch. Occup. Environ. Health*, **49**, 137–149.

Knauth P and Ilmarinen J (1975) Continuous measurement of body temperature during a 3-week experiment with inverted working and sleeping hours. In Colquhohn P, Folkard S, Knauth P and Rutenfranz J (eds) *Proceedings of the 3rd International Symposium on Night and Shiftwork*, 66–74. Westdeutscher Verlag.

Knauth P and Shonfelder E (1988) *Women and Nightwork*. Dublin: European Foundation.

Knutsson A (1989) Shift work and coronary heart disease. *Scandinavian Journal of Social Medicine*. Supplement 44.

Koller M (1989) Preventive health measures for shiftworkers. In Wallace M (ed.) *Managing Shiftwork*. Brain Behaviour Research Institute, 17–24. La Trobe University, Bundoora, Australia.

Lavie P (1986) Ultrashort sleep-waking schedule. 'Gates' and 'forbidden zones' for sleep. *Electroenceph. Clin. Neurophysiol.*, **63**, 414–425.

Lees R E M and Laundry B R (1989) Comparison of reported workplace morbidity in 8-hour and 12-hour shifts in one plant. *J. Soc. Occup. Med.*, **39**, 81–84.

Mott P E, Mann F C, McLoughlin Q and Warwick D P (1965) *Shiftwork: The Social, Psychological and Physical Consequences*. University of Michigan Press: Ann Arbor.

Pokorski J, Iskra-Golec I, Czekaj M and Noworol C (1990) Menstrual rhythm and shiftwork interference – a subjective retrospective study. In Costa G, Cesana G, Kogi K and Wedderburn A (eds) *Shiftwork: Health, Sleep and Performance*, 125–131. Frankfurt Main: Peter Lang.

Reinberg A (1974) Chronobiology and nutrition. *Chronobiologia*, **1**, 22–27.

Robson M and Wedderburn A (1990) Women's shiftwork and their domestic commitments. In Costa G, Cesana G, Kogi K and Wedderburn A (eds) *Shiftwork: Health, Sleep and Performance*, 137–143. Frankfurt Main: Peter Lang.

Rutenfranz J, Haider M and Koller M (1985) Occupational health measures for nightworkers and shiftworkers. In Folkard S and Monk T H (eds) *Hours of Work – Temporal Factors in Work Scheduling*. New York: Wiley.

Singer G (1989) Women and shiftwork. In Wallace M (ed.) *Managing Shiftwork*, 25–48. Brain Behaviour Research Institute, La Trobe University, Bundoora, Australia.

Smith A P and Wilson M (1990) The effects of naps during night duty on the performance and mood of female nurses working in an intensive care unit. In Costa G, Cesana G, Kogi K and Wedderburn A (eds) *Shiftwork: Health, Sleep and Performance*, 147–153. Frankfurt Main: Peter Lang.

Stephan F and Zucker I (1972) Circadian rhythms in drinking behaviour and locomotor activity of rats are eliminated by hypothalamic lesions. *Proceedings of the National Academy of Science, USA*, **69**, 1583–1586.

Taylor P J and Pocock S J (1972) Mortality of shift and day workers 1956–68. *Br. J. Ind. Med.*, **29**, 201–207.

Teiger C (1984) Overmortality among permanent nightworkers: some questions about adaptation. In Wedderburn A and Smith P (eds) *Psychological Approaches to Night and Shift Work*. Edinburgh: Heriot–Watt University.

Todd C, Reid N and Robinson G (1989) The quality of nursing care on wards working eight and twelve hour shifts: a repeated measures study using the MONITOR index of quality of care. *Int. J. Nurs. Stud.*, **26**, 4, 359–368.

Uehata T and Sasakawa N (1982) The fatigue and maternity disturbances of night work women. *Journal of Human Ergology*, **11**, Suppl. 465–474.

Vener K J, Szabo S and Moore J G (1989) The effect of shift work on gastrointestinal (GI) function: a review. *Chronobiologia*, **16**, 421–439.

Verhaegen P, Cober R, De Smedt M, Dirkx J, Kerstens J, Ryvers D and van Daele P (1987) The adaptation of night nurses to different work schedules. *Ergonomics*, **30**, 1301–1309.

Walker J (1985) Social problems of shiftwork. In Folkard S and Monk T H (eds) *Hours of Work: Temporal Factors in Work Scheduling*. Chichester: Wiley.

Wedderburn A (1975) *Studies of Shiftwork in the Steel Industry*, 218–220. Edinburgh: Department of Business Organisation, Heriot-Watt University.

Wedderburn A (ed.) (1989) *Women and Nightwork, Bulletin of European Shiftwork Topics 2*. European Foundation for the Improvement of Working and Living Conditions.

Wever R A (1979) *The Circadian System of Man: Results of Experiments under Temporal Isolation*. New York: Springer.

Zulley J, Wever R A and Aschoff J (1981) The dependence of onset and duration of sleep on the circadian rhythm of rectal temperature. *Pflugers Archiv.*, **391**, 314–318.

The Morningness Questionnaire Scoring:

Questions 1, 2, 10, 17 and 18: (a)=5 (b)=4 (c)=3 (d)=2 (e)=1.
Questions 3, 8, 9, 13 and 15: (a)=4 (b)=3 (c)=2 (d)=1.
Questions 11 and 19: (a)=6 (b)=4 (c)=2 (d)=0.
Question 12: (a)=0 (b)=2 (c)=3 (d)=5.
Questions 4, 5, 6, 7, 14 and 16: (a)=1 (b)=2 (c)=3 (d)=4.

Chapter 9
A Quality Assurance Programme for Night Nursing
Fiona M Hicks

Introduction

The aim of this chapter is to provide an overview of quality assurance and to introduce a quality assurance programme developed by night nurses within one health authority. This programme included the development of a standard of care for promoting sleep for individual patients during their hospitalisation. The steps involved in the development of the standard are discussed and the standard is presented in appendix 1.

Quality Assurance

Definitions of quality assurance found in the literature are many and varied. Bittle (1970) defined it broadly as 'those activities and programmes intended to assure quality of care'. Williamson (1982) used an operational definition 'the measurement of the actual level of the service provided plus the efforts to modify when necessary the provision of these services in the light of the results of the measurement'. Hibbs (1990) defined quality assurance as 'the process of assessment in order to maintain/improve the quality of services . . . it is those efforts that are made to evaluate, improve deficiencies and ensure the quality of care'. Definitions of quality assurance share similarities in that they include the three elements of:

- identification of values, standards and criteria;
- measurement to determine if they have been achieved;
- action to realign actual and agreed levels of care.

These three elements reflect the three important areas for any nursing quality assurance programme that were identified by Lang and Clinton (1984). These were:

- the describing phase;

- the measuring phase; and
- the action phase.

The model used by Hibbs was based on the model of quality assurance by Lang (1976) as used by the American Nurses Association. Both are circular which is indicative of the continuous nature of the quality assurance process. The CHPU model shows how values are identified, from which standards and criteria are developed (Figure 9.1). The criteria are then measured by either existing tools or by tools developed specifically. Data from these measurements are used to interpret and to identify deficiencies. Actions are then proposed, selected and taken. A phase of evaluation occurs before the process repeats itself.

Quality is undoubtedly subjective so hence the need for agreed levels of excellence. Kendall and Kitson (1986) said that which constitutes a quality service must be 'negotiated between providers, recipients and those who provide the resources'. The merger of the varied quality perspectives held by this tripartite group enable the identification of deficiencies and corrective action to be taken.

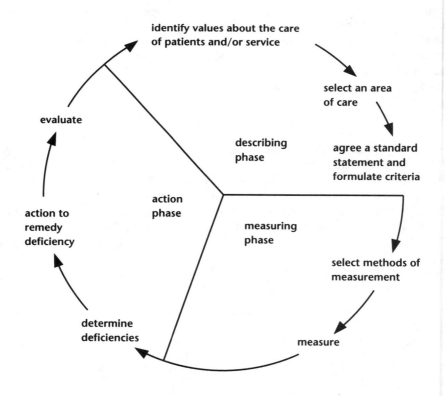

Figure 9.1 City and Hackney Praider Unit Model for Quality Assurance and Standard Setting (adapted from Lang 1976 and ANA 1982)

The Need for Quality Assurance in Health Care

Quality assurance has gained in stature in recent years. The reasons for this are multiple and encompass professional, consumer and political interests and also international and national advisory spheres.

Professional values form an important consideration when defining standards of care for patient groups. The United Kingdom Central Council for Nursing, Midwifery and Health Visiting (UKCC) documents *The Code of Professional Conduct* (clauses 1, 3, 10 and 11) and *Exercising Accountability* (Section B), have both addressed the maintenance of standards. Both of these documents make explicit and/or implicit references to the importance of the professional responsibility of nurses to define, monitor and ensure standards are not compromised. The Royal College of Nursing (RCN), concerned about the ability of its members to maintain an adequate standard of patient care, published two authoritative documents on setting, monitoring and evaluating standards of care within the nursing profession (RCN 1980, RCN 1981).

From a world-wide perspective the World Health Organisation's 'Health for all by 2000' (WHO 1984) in Target 31 stated that 'By 1990, all member states should have built effective mechanisms for ensuring quality of patient care within their health care systems'. This is a powerful advisory recommendation for all member states. As 1990 has passed and the year 2000 is rapidly approaching there is no room for complacency in relation to implementing quality assurance.

Increased consumer awareness has meant that patients are likely to be knowledgeable about the quality of service that should be provided. As the health service is funded by public money there is a social ethic created that value for money should pervade. Where organised consumer groups exist, these actively pursue and represent the interest of individual patients. Views of consumer expectations of a service must therefore be elicited. Documented evidence should be available which explicates the required and provided quality of a service. The quality needs to be measured and monitored.

Quality in health care in the United Kingdom has increasingly become a dominant issue. Griffith (1983), in addition to the reorganisation of the health service, made quality a major issue in health care management. Following the *Working for Patients* legislation (1991), which separated the purchasers of services from those providing the services, quality is high on the contractual agenda. Hospitals as 'Provider Units' will need to state the quality of service they will provide to the 'Purchasing Units'. Likewise, the 'purchasers' will be quick to stipulate the quality of service which they expect for their clients.

The Culture for Quality Assurance

A quality assurance drive should create an organisational climate which fosters change and innovation. A culture which lives and breathes total quality is the desired aim. A total quality service should regard every person or department that it interfaces with as a consumer and continually strive to provide it with the best service possible. Wilson (1987) emphasised that prerequisites for a quality assurance programme are the development of clear organisational goals and a well communicated value system which results in departmental philosophies, mission statements and goal setting. In CHPU nursing already had in place Wilson's (1987) prerequisites for a quality assurance programme. A district philosophy complemented by ward philosophies had been stated and annual objectives for nursing defined. The organisation had also stated its commitment to the provision of a quality service in its mission statement (Grant 1990). It thus seemed timely to initiate quality assurance programmes.

Nursing has, in general, moved to a problem-solving approach to quality assurance. This approach provides a local, realistic and practical method, which has been shown to be stimulating and meaningful for staff (Wilson 1987). This is reflected in a 'trend towards a unit based approach to quality assurance' (Harvey 1988). This approach has the benefit that it is 'owned' by the unit and thus will gain greater commitment, have greater relevance and be dynamic. This 'bottom-up' approach is consistent with the district quality assurance ethic as fostered by the organisation.

A Quality Assurance Programme Applied to Night Duty

Our quality assurance programme was started from an organisational perspective using Wilson's 'Adult Learning Model' (1987). It advocated the utilisation of existing data to initiate some quality monitoring and measurement. We were encouraged that many activities already in progress could be formalised into a quality assurance programme. Measurement was introduced to these and actions taken. It emphasised that quality assurance included many constituents and standards of care are only one part of a quality assurance programme. The quality assurance programme developed for night duty is shown in Figure 9.2. The constituents of each of the eight parts of this programme are expanded in Table 9.1. Nursing staff were permanent night staff and ward based nursing staff who rotated to night duty. Night sisters were unit based and rotated between units every 3 months. Other permanent night staff included staff nurses, enrolled nurses and auxiliaries.

The constituents of the programme were potentially general in nature. In implementing each constituent part, areas specific to night duty were used.

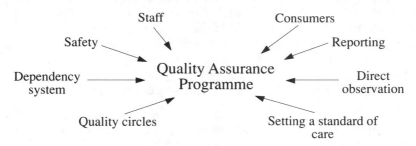

Figure 9.2   A Quality Assurance Programme for Night Duty

Table 9.1

The activities undertaken are shown in a list to give a flavour of the constituents of each part of the programme.

1. STAFF
- Register of qualification
- Checking agency staff qualification and personal identification number (PIN)
- Individual performance review
- Individual orientation programme
- Provision of training, education and professional development

2. CONSUMER
- Complaints policy
- Satisfaction survey (incorporated into standard outcome)

3. SAFETY
- Weekly survey of corridors
- Annual fire evacuation drill and twice yearly lecture
- Twice yearly resuscitation workshop

4. REPORTING
- Accidents/Incidents
- Untoward incidents
- Cross infections   Negative indicators reported to relevant clinical
- Pressure area sores   nurse specialists

5. DEPENDENCY STUDY/MANPOWER STUDY
- Financial Information Project (FIP)

6. DIRECT OBSERVATION AND LISTENING
- Gathering information informally from all staff and consumers

7. QUALITY CIRCLES
- A quality circle is a small group (4–10) of individuals who work together and who meet together voluntarily but formally and regularly to identify and solve work related problems in a systematic way. The night circle was composed of all grades of staff and led by a nurse trained in quality circle techniques.

8. SETTING A STANDARD OF CARE
- Several nursing quality assurance tools have either been imported into the UK or home grown in recent years. Each method has strengths and weaknesses and critiques of nursing QA tools pervade current literature. Nurses who are developing quality assurance packages should search out and assess the existing tools. Some of these have known levels of reliability and validity and will prevent wasted time and energy in developing new untested tools. An appraisal of the existing nursing quality measurement tools indicated that they did not address the provision of sleep for individual patients. The development of a programme to include a standard of care which provided for individual sleep needs in hospital seemed appropriate.

An example which related to safety was that on one random night every week items left in corridors were listed (equipment, furniture, rubbish, stores etc). This list was tabulated and each week copies were sent to all relevant departments including quality assurance, nurse managers, portering, risks department and domestic services. Actions taken to clear corridors included the allocation of an area for the return of portering wheel chairs and a designated storage area for ward beds which were temporarily out of use. The aim was to get some monitoring and quality improvement into place at an early stage to encourage staff.

A quality circle began in 1988 from a desire by nurses to address some of the problems experienced by night staff. An example of a problem identified and solved by the quality circle included ensuring adequate supply of linen for use at night. The stock of linen was often depleted before it was restocked at 08.00. An increase in the total stock level failed to solve this problem. The problem was solved by dedicating a back-up linen cupboard which was locked during the day. This resulted in an ample supply of linen being available to all wards throughout the night (and out of hours). Many more problems were solved by the use of the quality circle and this improved the quality of working life for staff and has made positive contributions to the quality of patient care.

Standard Setting for Nursing Care

Greene (1989) defined a standard as 'a professionally agreed level of perform-ance appropriate to the population addressed, which reflects what is observ-able, achievable, measurable and desirable care'. In that standards should be set at a level which is professionally desirable it is vital that nurses become involved in setting standards. It is the unique role of nurses which places them in a position to determine the standard of care given. Standards are needed to explicate what constitutes quality care. Nurses already have their individual standards internalised and use them to guide their practice. Stan-dard setting is an attempt to examine practice and clarify what groups of nurses agree to be quality nursing care for defined patient groups.

Standard Setting Method

'*The Dynamic Standard Setting System*' (RCN 1990), was the method used to guide standard setting in the Authority. It is a patient-centred approach to health care delivery and contains the elements of Williamson's (1971) problem-orientated approach and the structure, process and outcome domains from the Donabedian model (1986). These domains provide con-venient headings for grouping the criteria used in standard setting (see Table 9.2). The system, pioneered by Kitson (1989), viewed the practitioners as experts and considered that they are best equipped to set achievable standards of care. This is the 'bottom up' approach to quality assurance, an approach which still requires management commitment and leadership. Quality devel-opments were facilitated by one day workshops on standard setting and access to the clinical nurse specialist quality assurance as a resource person. Help was needed to clarify terminology, which was new and initially bewildering for us. This *Dynamic Standard Setting System* approach was valuable in

Table 9.2   Examples of criteria using the domains of structure, process and outcome

---

STRUCTURE

These criteria look at the setting in which the process of care takes place. They refer to the resources needed to accomplish the care that is:

- staff – number and skill mix
- staff knowledge
- availability of equipment and other facilities
- administrative and financial arrangements
- physical environment
- information

PROCESS

These criteria refer to the activities and interactions which staff perform to reach the standard that is:

- assessment techniques and procedures
- describing nursing actions in implementing and monitoring care
- methods of evaluation to be performed
- providing information to patients, relatives and carers
- providing education and training for patients, relatives and carers

OUTCOME

These criteria refer to the anticipated results of nursing care in relation to:

- patients' health status or behaviour
- patient and/or carers' knowledge
- patient and/or carers' level of satisfaction

---

guiding the development of the standard to provide for individualised sleep needs of patients (see Appendix 1 for the resultant standard of care and its audit tool).

Development of a Standard for Night Duty

This section gives an account of our experience in the development of the standard. It is divided into the three sections of describing, measuring and action which are used in the quality assurance cycle.

The Describing Phase   The nurses involved in this 'quality drive' believed in the therapeutic value of sleep and the unique role and expertise of night nurses. They sought to increase their knowledge by formulating a teaching programme which educated them about the nature, structure and function of sleep. A 'sleep' folder was created which contained relevant articles, research and information. This was used as a resource to aid teaching.

Reference to nursing research had indicated that patients were exposed to reduced total sleep time and disturbed sleep for many reasons. These reasons related to both the patients' condition and the environment. The late settling time (Bentley et al 1977, Dodds 1980) and the early wakening time (Bentley et al 1977, Stead 1985) were cited as reasons for reducing patients' amount of sleep. Dodds (1980) noted that patients 'once woken they may not have access to their usual remedy to restore sleep'. Walker (1972) and Woods

(1972) both found that post-operative patients were subject to much sleep disturbance because of nursing interventions.

Noise had been reported by many researchers as a cause of sleep disturbance (Bentley et al 1977, Dodds 1980, Hinks 1984, Hilton 1985, Closs 1988, Irwin 1989). Ogilvie (1980) found that Nightingale design wards were significantly louder at night than the modern cubicled/partitioned wards. This had implications for our practice as many wards were of Nightingale design. Other research papers identified sources of noise and levels of noise in decibels. Pain and physical discomfort were found as major disturbances to sleep (Closs 1988).

An investigation of our current practice was initiated by a descriptive survey of the patients' night in hospital. This survey ascertained the pattern of patients' sleep and any nursing routine. Information collected included:

- time patients were settled;
- time lights were dimmed;
- time patients were woken;
- time of medicine rounds;
- time breakfast was served;
- time of observations; and
- other stated incidents which disturbed patients' sleep.

The results from this survey were analysed and areas were identified for improvement. These areas included wards leaving main lights on until midnight and turning them back on as early as 6am to start morning work which included serving breakfast. Sleep was also disturbed because patients were woken for six hourly medication which had been prescribed for 02.30, also for twice daily observation of vital signs at 06.00.

Two wards, initially, were asked to participate in the development of the standard. The standard setting group consisted of one night nursing officer, one night sister, two night pool nurses, the two ward sisters and ward staff nurses who rotated to night duty. Monthly meetings were agreed to be held for a duration of one hour. Difficulties were experienced in arranging meetings because of the difference in shift working hours between day and night staff. Occasionally meetings were held at 08.00 or 20.00 but generally they were held at 14.00.

It was essential that the night staff had participation from the named wards involved in standard setting. Change cannot be introduced successfully without the need for change being accepted by all concerned. It was vital to consider the implication of any change on all staff and patients within each 24-hour day and not just between 22.00 and 07.00. An example of the importance of gaining both day and night perspectives on the same situation was illustrated by the time at which breakfast was served. Breakfast was served by the night staff so that the morning nursing activities could be readily accommodated. To delay breakfast would thus have an impact on the morning shift. The fact that breakfast was served when a minimum number of nurses were on duty begged the question of who was available to feed dependent patients. Breakfast trays were removed by domestics during morning handover, therefore nurses were unable to assess the amount and type of food eaten by patients. Situations, like this triggered lively debates about what constituted quality nursing and how this could be delivered.

To start on standard setting we compiled six broad value statements which related directly to the provision of sleep for individual patients (Table 9.3). This proved to be a beneficial starting point as it committed our values to paper. These statements were readily debated and from them a standard statement and the rudiments of criteria were written. The headings of structure, process and outcome were used to group the criteria. Criteria were formulated from research, our knowledge, professional guidelines, local policies, experience and practice. Many of the criteria were already part of normal nursing practice and this helped us realise that standard setting was making explicit what we do, why we do it and what we hope to achieve by our actions. Standard setting enabled us to identify good practice and to identify wards where this was already partially or wholly in practice. Ideas and values were shared and achievable criteria established. As the criteria were written those which were new to our practice were introduced to all staff. Gradually changes which included turning patients' bed lights on at 21.30 and dimming the main ward lights became part of our established practice. The night nursing staff wanted to ensure that everything possible would be done to provide for the individual sleep needs of each patient.

Table 9.3 Six broad value statements composed by the standard setting group

1. The staff will have knowledge and understanding of the therapeutic value of sleep in both physical and psychological well-being.

2. Each patient will have an individual assessment which includes assessment of usual sleep habits, identified needs and problems will have nursing actions documented on the care plan. A sleep evaluation will be documented.

3. The staff will manage the ward environment at night so that it is conducive to promoting maximum sleep.

4. Interruptions to sleep for therapeutic purposes will be minimised when possible. This can be achieved by such actions as clustering nursing actions together, assessing patients' condition and reappraising frequency of observations.

5. Nurses will facilitate, whenever possible, the patient to perform his or her usual pre-sleep routine and enable the patient to settle and rise when they wish.

6. The staff will provide a safe and comfortable environment.

The Measuring Phase   An audit tool is necessary to judge if a standard is being achieved. The standard is a statement related to the expected performance level and criteria are the individual variables to be appraised. Criteria thus operationalise the standard in terms of measurable quantitative guidelines. Audit tools should be written in conjunction with criteria, so that a method to measure each criterion is identified. Wilson (1987) suggested the mnemonic RUMBA to guide the writing of criteria, this reflects the need to ensure that they are measurable. He suggested that criteria should be:

R – relevant
U – understandable
M – measurable
B – behaviourally described
A – achievable.

The audit tool used should be valid and reliable. Polit and Hungler (1985) defined validity as the 'degree to which an instrument measures what it is supposed to measure' and reliability as the 'degree of consistency or dependability with which an instrument measures the attribute it is designed to measure'.

The audit tool is used to measure if the criteria and hence the standard has been achieved. Methods of measurement include:

- direct observation and information seeking;
- consumer satisfaction – interview/questionnaire;
- staff satisfaction – interview/questionnaire;
- documentation and chart audit;
- microbiological analysis;
- objective environmental measurements (temperature, noise etc);
- analysis of incident/accident forms; and
- reference to existing quality audit tools (monitor, qualpacs etc.)

Measurement can be concurrent or retrospective. Concurrent measurement takes place while care is still in progress whereas retrospective measurement occurs after the delivery of care is completed.

Consideration to the number of staff and the amount of time needed to perform an audit should be made. Consideration should also be given to who will perform the audit. Current thinking emphasises the concept of peer review (Pearson 1987). Peer review is 'a process by which practitioners of the same rank, profession or setting critically appraise each other's work performance against established standards' (O'Loughlin and Kaulback 1981). For example ward sisters would reciprocate for each other. This has the value of removing any punitive type fears that wards may have if audited by those in the hierarchy. Arguably those currently in practice are best equipped to perform audit as they are both practice and reality focused. Judging the quality of nursing care is a professional issue and one which nurses must perform.

The method of measurement most appropriate to the criteria being audited should be used. It is suggested that patients and staff should not be over-exposed to questionnaires. Over-exposure may result in apathy and poor response rate. Skill is needed in questionnaire design. Caution is needed when drawing conclusions from the responses since patients are generally reluctant to criticise the service and/or the care received (French 1981). They may also fear the 'threat of sanctions' (Rosso 1984). In quality assurance it is however, important to gather consumer opinion.

To audit the criteria in the night standard the following methods of measurement were selected:

- patients' opinions;
- direct observation of nursing practice;
- review of documentation;
- objective methods to measure environmental noise and temperature.

Patients' opinions were obtained using a 'likert-type' scale checklist (see Appendix 1). Analysis of this was simple and it produced adequate data for the purpose of audit. The checklist was easy for patients to complete. A sound meter was borrowed from the Risks Department to obtain a base line level of noise on the wards at night and thermometers were used to measure ward temperature.

It was considered reasonable to perform the audit at six monthly intervals. The frequency at which to audit will often depend on the topic/subtopic of the standard. The findings on audit were written up in a brief report and recommendations for action made. The working party decided not to use points or a scoring system. It was felt that it was most important for areas of concern to be indicated and actions implemented to rectify these rather than numerical scores being given.

The audit tool was piloted to test that it was effective and useable. Following the pilot test, alterations to the audit tool were made. Some compliance ratings were altered. Compliance is the level of expected conformality to the criteria being measured. The pilot showed that compliance of 100 per cent or 90 per cent as not achievable for some criteria due to extraneous variables – these were rewritten as 75 per cent. This is exemplified by noise levels on wards at night. The EEC recommended maximum for noise in bedroom areas at night is 35 decibels. It was shown on the pilot test that ward noise never dropped below a baseline of 45 decibels at night. The audit tool therefore needed to use 45 decibels as a baseline to make the standard realistic and achievable.

The Action Phase   The results of the audit identified deficits in the actual quality of care against the determined criteria. Areas for action are thus identified. An example of this is demonstrated in the action taken in relation to a source of noise at night. The skip into which materials for incineration are disposed, was located next to a ward block and was replaced three times a week in 'the middle of the night'. This policy had been agreed as acceptable because the large skip lorry had difficulty negotiating the busy congested narrow roads around the hospital. Data was collected regarding the times the lorry arrived and the disturbance it caused to patients' sleep. This was presented to management with proposed solutions. As a consequence the skip contractors were informed that the skips could not be exchanged between 21.00 and 07.00. This 'agreement' is prone to the occasional lapse and thus needs continual reinforcing. This negotiation involved liaising with several different departments in the hospital which is evidence that standard setting is often appropriately a multi-disciplinary endeavour. On such occasions the commitment of the whole organisation to providing a quality service is put to the test.

A further example is that four times daily antibiotics were often prescribed for 02.30. This principally occurred because the drug chart was designed around the six hourly times of 08.30, 14.30, 20.30 and 02.30 with gaps between these pre-printed times for hand written time requests. Visually the charts suggest to the prescriber that the pre-printed times should be used. Attempts to educate each set of prescribers not to prescribe routine medications at 02.30 have had limited success. The consequence is that proposals are under way to re-design the patient medication chart. These are a few examples of how the action phase can be used widely to improve the quality of care.

When setting standards for nursing care caution is necessary because many intervening variables impose on the outcome of nursing care. In many situations the patients themselves, the organisation, other health care workers or relatives may have an impact on the outcome. Outcome measurements in nursing are indeed an area requiring further development as they are very complex. Some outcome measures alone are too simplistic to measure the quality of nursing care. As nursing is a practice discipline the observation of process is of great importance.

Conclusion

This chapter has shown how the development of a quality assurance programme, which included setting a standard of care for patient sleep at night, improved the quality of care for patients. Quality assurance programmes can be started simply and built upon. Staff value the opportunity to describe what they, as professionals and experts, believe to be quality care. Standard setting empowers staff to take the initiative and make quality care a reality. Making explicit agreed, defined and measurable levels of quality is increasingly becoming an area in which nurses must be active.

References

American Nurses' Association and Sutherland Learning Ass. (1982) *Professional Nurses; Role in Quality Assurance, Nursing Quality Assurance Management Learning System* (vol 2). Kansas City, Missouri: American Nurses' Association.

Bentley S, Murphy F and Dudley H (1977) Perceived noise in surgical wards and an intensive care unit: an objective analysis. *British Medical Journal*, 10 Dec, 2, 6101, 1503–1506.

Bittle L (1970) In Wilson C (1987) *Hospital Wide Quality Assurance: Models of Implementation and Development*. Philadelphia: W B Saunders.

Clark J (1984) In Pearson A (ed.) (1987) *Nursing Quality Measurement: Quality Assurance Methods for Peer Review*. Chichester: John Wiley and Sons.

Closs S J (1988) *A Nursing Study of Sleep on Surgical Wards*. University of Edinburgh.

Donabedian A (1986) Criteria and standards for quality assessmsent and monitoring. *Quality Review Bulletin*, 12, 99–108.

Dodds E J (1980) *Slept Well? A study of ward activity and nurse-patient interaction at night*. Unpublished MSc Thesis University of Surrey.

French K (1981) Methodological considerations in hospital patient opinion surveys. *International Journal of Nursing Studies*, **18**, 7–32.

Grant K (1990) *Application for NHS trust status for services run by City and Hackney Health Authority*. The district management board. The NHS review group City and Hackney Health Authority.

Greene W (1989) Setting standards. *Surgical Nurse*, April, 24–6.

Griffith R (1983) *The Griffith Report*, Department of Health and Social Security, NHS management enquiry, HMSO.

Hagen F (1978) *Conceptual issues in appraising quality of nursing care*. Canada: Columbia University Teaching College, Columbia University Press.

Harvey G (1988) More tools for the job. *Nursing Times*, **84**, 24, 33–34.

Hibbs P J (1990) *Strategy for quality*. City and Hackney Praider Unit.

Hilton B A (1985) Noise in acute patient care areas. *Research in Nursing and Health*, **8**, 283–291.

Hinks M D (1984) *The Most Cruel Absence of Care*. London: Kings Fund.

Irwin H P (1989) *A comparative study of the self reported sleep patterns of medical patients on nightingale wards with and without partitions*. MSc Thesis, University of Manchester.

Kendall H and Kitson A (1986) Quality Assurance. *Nursing Times*, August 27.

Kitson A (1989) A theoretical framework for quality assurance – a patient centred approach to quality assurance in health care, Standards of Care Project. London: RCN.

Lang N (1976) Issues in quality assurance in nursing. In American Nurses' Association (eds) *Issues in Evaluation Research*. Kansas City, Missouri: American Nurses' Association.

Lang N and Clinton J (1984) Quality assurance – the idea and its development in the United States. In Willis L and Linwood M (eds) (1984) *Measuring the Quality of Nursing Care*. Edinburgh: Churchill Livingstone.

Ogilvie A (1980) Sources and levels of noise on the ward at night. *Nursing Times*, 31 July.

Pearson A (1987) *Nursing Quality Measurement: quality assurance methods for peer review*. Chichester: John Wiley and Sons.

O'Loughlin E L and Kaulbach D (1981) Peer review: a perspective for performance appraisal. *Journal of Nursing Administration*, 22 September.

Polit D and Hungler B (1985) *Essentials of Nursing Research*. USA: Lippincott.

Rosso M (1984) Knowledge of practice. In Willis L and Linwood M (eds) (1984) *Measuring the Quality of Nursing Care*. Edinburgh: Churchill Livingstone.

Royal College of Nursing (1980) *Standards of Nursing Care*. London: RCN.

Royal College of Nursing (1981) *Towards Standards*. London: RCN.

Royal College of Nursing (1989) *A theoretical framework for quality assurance – a patient centred approach to quality assurance in health care*. Standards of Care Project. London: RCN.

Royal College of Nursing (1990) *Dynamic Standard Setting System*, London: RCN.

Stead W (1985) One awake, all awake. *Nursing Mirror*, **160**, 16, 20–21.

United Kingdom Central Council for Nursing, Midwifery and Health Visiting (1984) *Code of Professional Conduct: A UKCC Document*. London: UKCC.

United Kingdom Central Council for Nursing, Midwifery and Health Visiting (1989) *Exercising Accountability: A UKCC Document*. London: UKCC.

Walker B (1972) The postsurgery heart patient: amount of uninterrupted time for sleep and rest during the first, second and third post-operative days in a teaching hospital. *Nursing Research*, **21**, 2.

Williamson J (1971) Evaluating the quality of patient care: a strategy relating outcome and process assessments. *Journal of American Medical Association*, **218**, 564–569.

Williamson J (1982) *Teaching Quality Assurance and Cost Containment in Health Care*. London: Jossey-Bass.

Wilson C (1987) *Hospital Wide Quality Assurance: Models for implementation and development*. London: W B Saunders.

Woods N (1972) Patterns of sleep in post cardiotomy patients. *Nursing Research*, **21**, July/Aug, 347–352.

World Health Organisation (1984) Basic documents (34th edn). Geneva: World Health Organisation.

Appendix One

Included in this appendix is the standard of care and audit tool developed to measure and assure the quality of care for patients at night.

The criteria used to quantify quality care are grouped under the headings of structure, process and outcome.

The audit tool states how criteria can be measured. The Likert-type scale patient satisfaction checklist is included as an example of one of the measurement tools devised and used.

STANDARD OF CARE FOR PATIENTS AT NIGHT

Topic: Sleep at night
Sub Topic: Environment and nursing activities
Care Group: Patients on Ward X
Compiled By: The working party for night standard 1989–1990
Achieved By: December 1989
Review Date: 6 monthly following each audit

STANDARD STATEMENT

Nurses will take account of patients' individual needs for sleep and ensure that the environment and nursing activities at night on ward X promote maximum sleep.

RATIONALE

The provision of adequate sleep for individual patients is an important part of nursing care. Sleep has therapeutic value to patients because it has both physical and mental restorative properties (Hayter 1980, Horne 1983, Adams and Oswald 1984).

References

Adams and Oswald (1984) Sleep helps healing. *Brit. Med. Journal*, **289**, 1400–1401.

Hayter (1980) The rhythm of sleep. *American Journal of Nursing*, March, 457–459.

Horne (1983) Mammalian sleep function with particular reference to man. In Mayers A (ed.) *Sleep Mechanism and Functions in Humans and Animals*. Van Nostrand Reinhold (UK).

STRUCTURE CRITERIA

1. When empty beds are available admissions at night will go to the Admissions Ward, to prevent disturbance in the main ward.

2. The ward will have a minimum staffing level of 2 nurses per night shift, one of which will be a ward staff nurse on internal rotation or a night pool staff nurse. The provision of staff will be calculated on patient dependency.

3. The nurse has access to:
   a) literature on circadian sleep-wake rhythms (e.g. Canavan 1986, Turpin 1986, Wardle 1986);
   b) research based literature on sleep disturbance at night (e.g. Whitfield 1975, Hilton 1985, Ogilvie 1980, Goodemote 1985, Closs 1988a, 1988b);
   c) literature regarding the physiology, psychology and functions of sleep (e.g. Canavan 1986, Turpin 1986, Wardle 1986)
   d) The British National Formulary.

4. The nurse will have knowledge of night sedations, their actions, side effects and contra-indications by:
   a) naming 3 drugs commonly used as night sedation;
   b) naming 3 side effects of night sedation;
   c) naming 2 clinical conditions that contra-indicate giving a patient night sedation.

5. The nurse will have a knowledge and understanding of the therapeutic value of sleep in recovery and well being. The nurse will demonstrate this knowledge by:
   a) identifying 3 beneficial effects of sleep;
   b) identifying 3 problems likely to be related to sleep deprivation.

6. The window blinds/curtains:
   a) cover the whole window;
   b) are light occlusive;
   c) are in working order.

7. Every bed has an individual light which is in working order and sited in an appropriate position.

8. All telephones and call bells must have a mute facility and working light signal.

9. Curtains around patients' beds are:
   a) opaque;
   b) fully occlusive;
   c) can be drawn quietly.

10. When faults occur with bed lights, night lights, blinds, TV ear pieces etc., requests for repairs will be made within 24 hours. The repairs should be carried out within 5 working days if the parts are available.

11. There is equipment available to enable the nurse to moderate the ambient temperature i.e. working radiator valves, extra heaters/fans, extra blankets, means of opening or closing windows.

References

Canavan (1986) The functions of sleep. *Nursing*, **9**, 321–324.

Closs (1988a) Patients' sleep wake rhythms in hospital (Part 1). *Nursing Times*, Occasional paper, Vol 84, No 1.

Closs (1988b) Patients' sleep wake rhythms in hospital (Part 2). *Nursing Times*, Occasional paper, Vol 84, No 2.

Goodemote (1985) Sleep deprivation in the hospitalised patients. *Orthopaedic Nursing*, Vol 4, No 6, 33–35.

Hilton (1985) Noise in acute patient care areas. *Research in Nursing and Health*, Vol 8, 283–291.

Ogilvie (1980) Sources and levels of noise on the ward at night. *Nursing Times*, 31 July 1980.

Turpin (1986) Psychophysiology of sleep. *Nursing*, **9**, 313–319.

Wardle (1986) The chronology of sleep. *Nursing*, **9**, 325–326,

Whitfield (1975) Noise on the ward at night. *Nursing Times*, 13 March.

PROCESS CRITERIA

1. The nurse will ensure that interruptions to sleep for therapeutic purposes are kept to a minimum as long as it does not adversely affect the patient. This can be achieved in the following ways:
   a) By actively encouraging 6 hourly medicines to be prescribed at: 0600, 1200, 1800 and 2400 thereby not waking patients at 02.30 for medicines. The 24.00 medicines can be dispensed on settling patient for the night and 06.00 given as patient wakes up. (It is accepted that the drugs given more frequently must continue to be given through the night.)
   b) By reducing the frequency of nursing observations whenever the clinical condition of the patient permits; and if the patient requires frequent nursing interventions the timing of these should be planned by the nurse to take place at one sleep interruption, rather than intermittently.
   c) By deferring to day-time routine non-urgent treatment which requires frequent sleep interruptions for nursing observations (e.g. non-urgent blood transfusions).

2. the nurse will create an environment at night to promote sleep between the hours of 2200 and 0700 by:
   a) turning down the main ward lights by 2130 (in summer the blinds will be closed by 2130);
   b) not opening blinds or turning on main lights until 0700;
   c) reducing noise to a minimum;
   d) regulating the environmental temperature and ventilation to maintain patients' comfort (18–21C).

3. Each patient has their individual sleep needs assessed.

4. Each patient is encouraged to maintain their usual pre-sleep routine.

5. Any difficulties related to the provision of nursing care and/or facilitating sleep will be reported to the Night Sister/Charge Nurse overnight.

OUTCOME CRITERIA

1. On audit 75% of patients indicate their satisfaction with the environment for sleep in terms of:
   a) lighting –
      • ability to control own bed light
      • main lights off time
      • main lights on time
   b) noise level –
      • ward noise
      • noise from outside

   c) ambient temperature.

2. On audit 75% of patients are satisifed with the choices of methods to relax offered before sleep:
   a) hot drinks;
   b) pre-bed time relaxation routines;
   c) time of settling;
   d) and if necessary sleep medication.

3. 75% of patients are satisfied with:
   a) the amount of sleep obtained on the previous night;
   b) the time they woke this morning;
   c) the sleep they actually obtained in relation to the amount of sleep they expected to obtain.

4. 75% of patients state that they are satisfied with:
   a) the bed;
   b) the bedcovering;
   c) the adequacy of the pain control offered;
   d) the opportunity to discuss their anxieties with a nurse.

5. Only the number of patients identified as needing direct care will be disturbed during the process of care.

6. all patients are made comfortable in order that they may settle to sleep:
   a) their bed/bedding is prepared for the night
   b) all patients who needed assistance were positioned as comfortably as appropriate to their condition;
   c) patients liable to suffer pain had the appearance of being pain free and when asked stated this to be so.

7. Noise levels attributable to nurses will not exceed 45 decibels (the baseline measurement for Ward X), on testing with acoustic equipment.

8. There is evidence in all nursing records that patients' sleep needs have been assessed.

9. There is evidence in the nursing records of patients with assessed sleeping difficulties that sleep is identified as a problem on the care plan and goals set, actions implemented and the sleep pattern evaluated.

AUDIT TOOL FOR NIGHT STANDARD – STRUCTURE CRITERIA

Methods: direct observation and direct questions to staff. TICK appropriate response: when a NO response is recorded action will be needed.

1. No admission to ward overnight N/A if admissions ward fully occupied	YES NO NA
2. Minimum staffing level of two nurses one of whom is a ward staff nurse or night pool staff nurse	YES NO

3. Nursing literature on ward:
  a) Literature on circadian sleep-wake rhythms
    • Canavan 1986
    • Turpin 1986
    • Wardle 1986
	YES NO

b) Research-based literature on sleep disturbance at night
    • Whitfield 1975
    • Hilton 1976
    • Ogilvie 1980
    • Goodemote 1985
    • Closs 1988a
    • Closs 1988b
	YES NO

c) Literature on physiology, psychology and functions of sleep
    • Canavan 1986
    • Turpin 1986
    • Wardle 1986
	YES NO

d) British National Formulary	YES NO

4. Nursing knowledge of night sedations:
  a) 3 drugs commonly used as night sedation
  b) 3 side effects of night sedation
  c) 2 clinical conditions in which night sedation is contra indicated
	1 2 3
	1 2 3
	
	1 2

5. Nursing knowledge of the therapeutic value of sleep
  a) 3 beneficial effects of sleep
  b) 3 problems associated with sleep deprivation
	
	1 2 3
	1 2 3

6. Window blinds/curtains:
  a) cover all the window
  b) are light occlusive
  c) are in working order
	
	YES NO
	YES NO
	YES NO

7. Bed lights:
  a) Every bed has one
  b) All are placed within reach of patient
  c) All are in working order
	
	YES NO
	YES NO
	YES NO

8. Mute facility working:
  a) Telephone
  b) Call bells
	
	YES NO
	YES NO

9. Curtains around patients' beds:		
a) Opaque	YES	NO
b) Fully occlusive	YES	NO
c) Can be drawn quietly	YES	NO
10. Repairs pending (indicate date when requested):		
a) Bed lights	YES	NO
b) Night lights	YES	NO
c) Blinds	YES	NO
d) Other (state which) . . .		
11. Temperature control facilitated by		
a) Extra blankets	YES	NO
b) Fans available	YES	NO
c) Portable heaters	YES	NO
d) Radiator valves are in working order	YES	NO
e) Windows can be opened	YES	NO

AUDIT TOOL FOR NIGHT STANDARD – PROCESS CRITERIA
Methods

Question 1a: medication chart audit
Question 1b–2c: direct observation
Question 2d: check room thermometer reading
Question 3: documentation audit
Question 4: ask patient
Question 5: ask staff

1a. Routine 6 hourly medications are prescribed at 24.00, 06.00, 18.00 and 12.00 (not 02.30)	YES	NO
1b. Evidence that frequency of nursing observations are reduced at night	YES	NO
1c. Non-urgent treatments are postponed to day	YES	NO
2a. Ward blinds/main ward lights turned down by 21.30	YES	NO
2b. Ward blinds/main lights not turned up again until 07.00	YES	NO
2c. There is minimal noise from		
i) Staff talking	YES	NO
ii) Staff shoes	YES	NO
iii) Equipment	YES	NO
iv) Staff activity	YES	NO
2d. Environmental temperature is maintained between 18–21C and attempts are made to rectify extremes of temperature	YES	NO
3. Each patient has their individual sleep needs assessed	YES	NO
4. Each patient is encouraged to maintain their usual pre-sleep routine	YES	NO
5. Difficulties relating to the provision of care according to the standard are reported to the Night Sister/Charge Nurse	YES	NO

AUDIT TOOL FOR NIGHT STANDARD – OUTCOME CRITERIA
Methods
Question 1–5: patient checklist
Question 6a–c: direct observation
Question 6d: direct question
Question 7: noise measurement
Question 8 and 9: documentation audit

1. On audit 75% of patients indicated their satisfaction with the environment for sleep in terms of:	TICK
a) lighting	
• ability to control own bed light	YES NO
• lights off time	YES NO
• lights on time	YES NO
b) noise level	
• ward noise	YES NO
• noise from outside	YES NO
c) ambient temperature	YES NO
2. On audit 75% of patients were satisfied with the choices of methods to relax offered before sleep	YES NO
a) hot drinks	
• timing	YES NO
• choice	YES NO
b) pre-bed time relaxation routines	YES NO
c) time of settling	YES NO
d) and if necessary sleep medication	YES NO
3. 75% of patients were satisfied with the	
a) amount of sleep obtained last night	YES NO
b) the time you woke this morning	YES NO
c) the sleep you obtained last night in relation to the amount of sleep you expected to obtain	YES NO
4. 75% of patients state that they are satisfied with	
a) the bed	YES NO
b) the bedcovering	YES NO
c) the adequacy of the pain control	YES NO
c) the opportunity to express and discuss their anxieties with a nurse	YES NO
5. Only the number of patients identified as needing direct care will be disturbed during the process of care.	TICK INITIAL
A. No other patients disturbed	A.
B. 1–2 other patients disturbed	B.
C. 3–5 patients disturbed	C.
D. More than 5 other patients disturbed	D.

6. Patients were made comfortable in order that they may settle to sleep:
   a) Their bed/bedding was prepared for the night
      - A. more than 76%
      - B. 51–75%
      - C. less than 50%
   b) Were all patients who needed assistance positioned comfortable as appropriate to their condition
      - A. more than 76%
      - B. 51–75%
      - C. less than 50%
   c) Were patients liable to suffer pain have the appearance of being pain free
      - A. more than 76%
      - B. 51–75%
      - C. less than 50%
   d) Were patients liable to suffer pain able to state that they were pain free
      - A. more than 76%
      - B. 51–75%
      - C. less than 50%

7. Noise levels attributable to nurses do not exceed 45 decibels (the baseline measurement for Ward X), on testing with acoustic equipment
   - A. at any time during the night
   - B. on less than 5 occasions
   - C. on more than 6 occasions

8. There is evidence in all nursing records that patients' sleep needs have been assessed
   - A. In 100%
   - B. 76–99%
   - C. 51–75%
   - D. less than 50%

9. There is evidence in the nursing records of patients with assessed sleeping difficulties that sleep is identified as a problem on the care plan and goals set, actions implemented and sleep pattern evaluated
   - A. In 100%
   - B. 76–99%
   - C. 51–75%
   - D. less than 50%

A.
B.
C.

A.
B.
C.

A.
B.
C.

A.
B.
C.

A.
B.
C.

A.
B.
C.
D.

A.
B.
C.
D.

NIGHT TIME PATIENT SATISFACTION CHECKLIST   **CODE NO.**

Please tick the box which best describes the following aspects of your sleep last night

Item	Very satisfactory	Satisfactory	Unsatisfactory	Very unsatisfactory
1. Ability to control own bed light				
2. Time main lights turned off last night				
3. Time main lights turned on this morning				
4. Level of noise on the ward				
5. Level of noise from external source				
6. Ward temperature and ventilation			Too Hot Too Cold	Too Hot Too Cold
7. Time pre-bed drinks served				
8. Choice of pre-bed drinks				
9. The ease with which you could perform your usual pre-sleep routine				
10. The choice you had in the time you settled down to sleep last night				
11. Offer of sleeping tablet if desired				
12. The amount of sleep obtained on the previous night				
13. The time you woke this morning				
14. The sleep you actually obtained in relation to the amount of sleep you expected to obtain				
15. Bed				
16. Bedcovering				
17. Treatment measures to relieve pain or discomfort				
18. The opportunity to talk to a nurse at any time about things that worry you				

19. Were you woken by nurses attending to other patients?   YES
                                                                NO

20. Any other comments

Thank you for helping us improve our care to other patients

Chapter 10
The Education of Nurses Who Work at Night
Joan Kemp

The education of nurses who work at night is not often discussed in books and journals. Is this because they have no special educational needs? This chapter will address a number of issues that are central to the education of nurses who care for patients at night, with special reference to those who work permanently on the night shift. These include the need for information on the effects of night work, the difficulties of keeping up-to-date in matters relating directly to patient care, teaching student nurses at night, and professional development.

Setting the Scene

All nurses trained in Britain will recall their first experiences of night duty as pupil or student nurses. If they were trained before the mid-seventies, they may have spent as much as 25 per cent of their clinical training on night duty. Little attention was paid by senior nurses or tutors to the difficulties encountered by learners in adjusting from day work to night work or vice versa. Indeed, the way in which a learner coped with night duty was taken as a measure of his/her suitability for a career in nursing. Such a rite of passage was part of the apprenticeship to nursing and it contributed to wastage from the profession. Again, until the end of the seventies, it was common for staff nurses aiming for a post as ward sister or charge nurse to take a short-term appointment of about twelve months as a night sister for 'experience'. Older nurses reminiscing about these early experiences of night duty will remember being in charge of a hospital ward, sometimes alone, for long periods of the night. In contrast, the learners of today have freedom from responsibility; night duty is expected to be an educational experience under the supervision of qualified nurses who, in consequence, have a teaching role.

The atmosphere of a hospital, nursing home or residential unit at night is different from that in the day time. The larger the institution, the more marked is the difference. These are noisy places by day. Consider the sounds of activity coming from a kitchen, a bathroom, an entrance hall or an office.

Remember the telephone, the television set, visitors. The work of health care staff is guided by the constant exchange of information. Moreover, patients or residents inform, support and entertain each other through conversation. At night most of this ceases. The gradual fall in noise levels in a hospital or nursing home late in the evening is the signal to the night nurses that they will be reliant on their own resources. Stores are closed, fewer clinical experts are on hand to give advice, faulty equipment will not be repaired and the nurses take on the work of kitchen maid, porter and Jack of all trades. Resourcefulness and self-sufficiency are characteristics of night staff and they take pride in them. The price of long-term self-sufficiency may be high because it probably reinforces the night nurses' sense of isolation from those who work by day.

Let us now take two vignettes of a night nurse working as one of a trio of: qualified nurse, nursing auxiliary and student nurse. This is a typical team on hospital work at night. The following descriptions are relevant to other care settings too, as will be shown later.

Mrs White is a registerd nurse with thirteen years' experience of permanent night duty. She works three nights per week, always on the same ward and on the same nights as a nursing auxiliary who is a good friend and in whose judgement she has confidence. Most nights there is a student nurse, who must never be left without supervision by a qualified nurse. Mrs White prefers not to leave the ward at all during the night. She is an experienced and skilful nurse, accustomed to taking decisions on the care of gravely ill patients, to 'holding' situations when necessary and to advising sleepy doctors as to the options available. The nursing auxiliary is regarded as a trustworthy deputy who does not require constant supervision. Mrs White is wary of student nurses, fearing that their questions 'How?', 'Why?' 'What?' may expose some gap in her knowledge. This threat causes her to avoid situations where they might ask 'awkward' questions. Avoidance not only deprives students of opportunities to gain knowledge but it deprives Mrs White too and is stressful for all. Students find Mrs White formal and remote; they busy themselves about the ward and prefer to talk to the nursing auxiliary.

Mrs Baker is an enrolled nurse with eight years' experience of night duty. She does not wish to work on the day shifts while her children are still at school nor to study to become a registered nurse. She is in charge of her ward at least two nights per week, supervising various nursing auxiliaries or student nurses and is regarded as a highly competent nurse. Mrs Baker enjoys the constant change of staff: 'the students bring a breath of fresh air. It's easy to get into a rut on nights'. During quiet periods they discuss patient care problems or the students' objectives and search together for information from the ward bookshelf, learning from each other. Mrs Baker says: 'It's important that students realise you understand how they feel on night duty. If you've got someone who's nervous, they pass their anxiety on to the patient'. Students leave the ward with a positive view of night work, saying: 'You could ask the night staff anything. They always had time for you'.

These introductory descriptions of night duty will be familiar to nurses who have worked at night. Either they present personal experience or they apply to someone known to the reader. Some will sympathise with the predicament of Staff Nurse White, caught in a cycle of isolation and avoidance, while others will question the apparent lack of self development among permanent night nuses.

Readers could ask themselves:

1. How does my experience of night duty compare with the description above?
2. What impressions would a student nurse, or any newcomer to night duty, take away from the workplace at night?

Being Different

If one asks a nurse to describe the night shift, often the reply is that it is 'different', 'patients are different at night'. By this, nurses seem to imply that their patients *behave* differently at night. After all, the patient or resident is the same person, with the same strengths and deficits by night as by day, whether he/she is in a surgical ward or a nursing home, whether he/she is mentally ill or is being rehabilitated following a stroke. Among those receiving nursing care at night, there is a hard core of problems that is distinctive. The problems are pain, sleeplessness, anxiety and a sense of loneliness – and they are interrelated. Being a nurse is also essentially different at night. Not only is it abnormal to work at night, requiring conscious and sustained effort to maintain such an altered life-style but night nurses are on the periphery of the extensive health care team that is audibly and visibly most active by day.

In assessing the educational needs of nurses who work, or who eventually will work, at night, we need to take account of the following circumstances in their workplace:

- what proportion of the staff work both night and day shifts over a period of months?
- is there a permanent night shift?
- are individuals able to choose which shift(s) and hours they will work?
- how efficient is the network of communication between night staff and senior managers or educators?

There can be no justification for denying nurses on night duty equality with those on day duty when it comes to the provision of education facilities. There *is* discrimination on the grounds that night nurses work 'awkward hours' and are inaccessible or that they work *only* two nights per week. Worse is the defeatist excuse: 'the night staff aren't interested. . . .' Where there is suspicion of inequality of opportunity for what are often scarce resources, with permanent night staff most disadvantaged, the latter identify the following reasons for not taking up the facilities of a course, lecture, conference or demonstration:

- it is held at the wrong time;
- the notice is too short;
- the subject matter is irrelevant to night staff;
- the night staff are not invited;
- staffing levels are too low for nurses to change their nights on duty;
- nurse managers selectively filter invitations to attend;
- nurse managers discourage applications to attend.

Such were the perceptions of a group of permanent night nurses interviewed by Kemp (1989). The focus of their complaints were thus the nurse teachers who did not consider the special needs of night nurses and the nurse managers who coped with running a night nursing service on minimum staffing levels.

Education for Caring at Night

Preparing for Night Work

The education of nurses for caring at night ought to begin with caring for the well-being of the nurses themselves. Unfortunately, it is still rare to find a pre-registration syllabus that addresses the questions of shift work, night work, disturbed circadian rhythms and sleep patterns. It is more common for nurses in training to learn experientially about the effects of night work on their bodies and on their social lives. Thus a student may suffer gastro-intestinal disorder, for example, without realising that this is not uncommon among night workers. Those who become very tired may make serious errors of judgement or be unusually clumsy and may attribute their poor perform-ance at work to personal inadequacy. Irritability and low spirits, 'taking it out' on friends and relatives, is another consequence of a bad night or a bad day's sleep. It is not helpful to tell a student new to night duty that if he or she has ever attended an all-night party, the night shift and its after-effects will be no problem. After all, few of us have to attend four all-night parties in a row!

Nurses who are about to go on night duty for the first time would benefit from information on the effects of night work and advice on coping strategies. Those who work regularly at night, especially permanent night nurses, need the opportunity to discuss in a structured way the longer-term effects of night work on themselves and their family. This book is intended to contribute to just such forward-looking discussion.

Informed Choice

Employers have a responsibility to help their staff to adjust to night work by providing them with ways and means to discuss abnormal hours of work. Nurses' choice of night work would then be *informed* choice. Night work would not be compulsory. At present, the choice is limited; nurses in training are required to gain a brief experience of patient care at night in hospital. It is also still the case in some localities that the night shift is unpopular and as much of a problem as it was in 1958, when the Royal College of Nursing reported on 'The Problem of Providing a Continuous Nursing Service Especially in Relation to Night Duty' (Royal College of Nursing 1958). Newly-qualified nurses may be offered the 'choice' between night duty or no work at all. Education for choice of shift is an ideal towards which far-sighted employers would be wise to move; there is a relationship between hours of work, job satisfaction and commitment to the constraints of the shift.

Keeping Up-to-Date with Developments in Nursing Care

We scarcely notice how much information we absorb in our daily lives: at work in a hospital or nursing home one learns to plan for changes within the institution and of new developments in the treatment of illness, for example, in diagnostic techniques, drugs, dressings and equipment. The information is sometimes from a secondary source but documents, directives and product brochures are available for the asking. The innovator may even be there in person to explain the latest development. Informal learning about patient care goes on all the time – it is facilitated by hand-over reports, case conferences, lunch and coffee breaks and occurs even in the staff changing room. This applies to doctors and therapists as well as the nurses. The nurses who work on the night shift for months or years at a stretch are at a disadvantage in this informal information exchange. Like Mrs White (page 15) some meet only two or three other nurses and a busy, tired doctor in the course of their eleven hours of work. In a small residential care unit, there may be no other qualified nurse present. After a few weeks of working on the night shift, the staff begin to realise that their information is sometimes third hand and altered along the way, as in the game of 'Chinese Whispers'.

It is a common complaint of night staff that discussion of patient care at the turn of shift *excludes* rather than encourages the contribution of the night nurse. If ownership of the plan of care, of the process of nursing, seems to be vested in the day staff, night nurses may well set such written plans aside for the night and leave them in the office. This is evidence that ten years after the introduction of the nursing process in British hospitals, it was not necessarily applied at night. The results of a large-scale investigation of night nursing services, involving a representative sample of 40 District General Hospitals and 796 nurses, were published in 1987 (National Health Service Management Consultancy Services 1987). The resultant nursing activity profile showed that 'the organisation of work at night seemed to a significant extent to be based on historic patterns over which the introduction of the nursing process has had little influence'. Adherence to those 'historic patterns' of task-orientated care was attributed to two deficiencies in the night nursing services: first, to a lack of qualified nurses and over-reliance on unqualified staff and, secondly, to *the lack of involvement of night staff* in the development of new systems of nursing care.

Nurses on permanent night duty are disadvantaged in their efforts to keep up-to-date by the nature of their work. Their aim is that patients should obtain as good a night's sleep as possible. Nursing interventions should therefore be at a minimum. Thus, night nurses apply fewer dressings and bandages, administer a narrower range of drugs and carry out fewer procedures in general than do their day time colleagues. Inevitably, they handle fewer products and less equipment, yet *they must be prepared* to use those items not normally handled for, one night, the need will arise. Less familiarity creates uncertainty, especially when faced with new products already familiar to those who care for patients by day. The problem of maintaining their skills and knowledge in the tasks of patient care is a serious one for nurses on long-term night duty and is a cause of considerable embarrassment for many of them. The skills in which experienced night nurses excel, comfort measures for sleepless and anxious patients, fortunately do not date but grow with experience.

Nurses on night duty develop a number of survival techniques to counteract the isolation of their working environment. One such strategy is to establish a 'hotline' to day-time practice by relying on a well-informed friend on the day shifts to relay useful information into their own home when both are off duty. Another valued resource is the hospital night sister, or the manager of night-time services, whose business it is to be well-informed about patient care twenty-four hours a day, for they bridge the gap between night and day shifts. A third survival technique, which is not often acknowledged, is to consult a second or third-year student nurse on the latest developments in wound dressings, incontinence garments or pain charts. Readers will remember Mrs White and Mrs Baker (pages 150–1) who reacted differently to students. Kemp (1989), in her study of a group of night nurses, found that the teaching function of learners was of value to the nurses.

In units where night and day staff are regarded equally as members of a twenty-four hour care team, the nurses on night duty are involved in the assessment of patients' (or residents') capabilities and problems. They are experts on strategies for helping patients to sleep and to cope with pain. They contribute to rehabiliation. Care plans for patients, or residents, are made in consultation with the night staff and preparations for discharge cannot proceed without a report from the night nurse. In such an atmosphere of collaboration – and it is possible where there is a permanent night shift as well as in a system of internal relation of staff – learning will be pain-free.

The teaching of night nurses, at night, about patient care is usually the task of a named individual in a hospital or other institution. It is often a night sister or ward sister/charge nurse with an aptitude for teaching or a nurse teacher who is willing to work at night. With low levels of staffing, much of the teaching and learning is on a one-to-one basis and opportunist, but a rolling programme of demonstrations and topics for discussion does much to boost the confidence of nurses on permanent night duty. The teachers themselves must be sustained by enthusiastic day-time contacts if they are not to flag because they too can become very isolated.

Protracted night duty leads to loss of confidence and 'know how', which must be recognised by employers and nurse managers for what it is: an occupational hazard among night nurses. They have a responsibility to alleviate this.

Preparation for Teaching and Supervising Students at Night

It is important that experience of the care of sick and frail people at night will continue to form part of the student nurse's curriculum. Without this experience, pre-registration education would not be complete. That there is much to learn from working at night is shown by the topics covered in this book.

The time spent by learners on night duty is greatly reduced today and may be no more than one or two weeks. When the learner arrives with precise learning objectives to be met in a short, single allocation to night duty, the quality of the supervision provided by the registered, or first level, nurse is crucial. Neither Mrs White nor Mrs Baker, who were described earlier, entirely fulfil that role. We must also bear in mind that the demands made on an individual qualified nurse at night are great. Staffing levels at night are unlikely to increase in the near future; registered nurses will continue to care for patients, teach students and manage the ward simultaneously with support from unqualified staff.

One of the aims of student nurses on night duty nowadays is to observe and participate in the care of patients they have already nursed by day. Thus they witness a twenty-four hour cycle of care. It is essential that their objectives for a brief, concentrated spell of night duty be drawn up in consultation with the nurses who staff the wards at night and not by nurse teachers alone. Few nurse teachers work at night and they are likely to have as many misconceptions about night work as permanent night nurses have about the day shift!

It is already common practice for experienced registered nurses to undertake a course in teaching and assessing students. Mentorship or preceptorship are becoming familiar terms. Nurses who work on permanent night duty are poorly represented on teaching courses but the reasons for this are unclear. Do night nurses find teaching courses irrelevant because they focus on day-time activities? Do course organisers see their courses irrelevant because they focus on day-time activities? Do course organisers see their courses as irrelevant to night nurses because teaching and assessing do not occur at night? Permanent night nurses do have great difficulty in obtaining the practical experience of assessment that is necessary for completion of a course. One cannot escape the conclusion that internal rotation favours the clinical nurse with a teaching function. The permanent night nurse who cannot obtain at least a short day-time work experience of, say, four to six weeks, is at a decided disadvantage.

The Professional Development of Night Nurses

Whereas much that has been said so far on education is, in part, the responsibility of a nurse's employer, continuing professional development is not.

Professional development is coping with change, entering and contributing to the debate on change and taking a long-term view of the nursing profession. Recent examples that come to mind are the role of the nursing assistant in relation to that of the qualified nurse and the increasing emphasis on the role of the nurse in health education. Professional development is not simply about reading the weekly nursing journals and attending a lecture or conference, though these are important too. Nurses must take an interest in the work of other health care professionals, in social policy, in local politics and in the results of health care research. This is the ideal that is easier to prescribe than to practise!

The reality is that irregular and unsocial hours of work, in particular lengthy periods of night work, seem to inhibit the professional development of many nurses. Permanent night nurses, who are mainly women with dependent children, suffer disordered circadian rhythms and chronic fatigue which are not conducive to self-directed learning.

Professional development is not synonymous with career progression and promotion. Not everyone wishes to change posts regularly or to be promoted but this does not imply a lack of intellectual curiosity. Night nurses often set aside earlier career plans for ten to fifteen years, while they bring up a family. Sadly, when they feel free to branch out and to apply for a new post, they discover that their experience of night duty counts for little in competition with nurses who have remained on day duty. Moreover, a 'professionally-underdeveloped' night nurse reinforces the prejudice that night staff in general are distinterested in continuing education. Thus the vicious circle continues (Kemp 1989).

The nurse who is registered to practise has an obligation to demonstrate that that practice is underpinned by continuous professional self-development. The two quotations that follow highlight its importance.

As Registrar and Chief Executive of the United Kingdom Central Council for Nursing, Midwifery and Health Visiting (UKCC), Maude Storey (1986) stated:

> the individual nurse, upon re-registration, will need to demonstrate that she has taken the opportunity to maintain and improve her own knowledge and skills allied to practice. This does not simply refer to attendance at readily available courses, and the broad deployment of valuable resources. The individual nurse will need to take responsibility for her own professional develpment.

In their book on ethics in health care, Downie and Calman (1987) write:

> it is quite common for professional carers to live a life of devotion to their patients as a result of which their own lives become empty and impoverished. They have cultivated only their medical knowledge and skills and have nothing to say on anything else. The duty of self-development can also be justified in terms of its benefit to other people. Since so much of the success of a doctor, nurse, dentist or other health worker depends on

the relationship each has with a patient, and since the nature of that relationship depends partly on the patient's perceptions of his helper, it is vital that the professional should be seen as an authentic human being who happens to be a doctor, nurse or other carer. If a doctor [or nurse] is to give himself to others he must have something to give!

Self-development, then, benefits nurses on several levels: it is recommended for periodic re-registration to practise, it is satisfying in itself and it enriches the nurse's relationships with patients or clients. By extension, the nurse's colleagues benefit too, as do any students with whom he or she comes into contact. What seems to be lacking is a culture, or an expectation, that professional development is as necessary to permanent night nurses as it is to all other qualified staff who work on permanent day shifts or on internal rotation to night duty.

Fixed and therefore predictable hours of work are a persuasive factor in the decision to work on the night shift. They allow paid work to be dovetailed with domestic activities. Most female night nurses manage their off-duty time with great precision and develop a Box and Cox arrangement whereby there is always someone (a family member) at home to look after small children while the mother is at work, or sleeping. This ability to manage time suggests that 'reading time' or 'professional time' could also be accommodated in the week's schedule. Making space in one's life for personal enrichment can arouse feelings of guilt.

When a nurse first takes up long-term night work the *expectation* that he or she will continue to learn needs to be expressed firmly and clearly. Even then some aims should be formulated. Continuing education facilities must be available, of course, and accessible to night nurses. A creche for young children might be an added encouragement.

Special programmes of education for night staff, unless dealing with specific aspects of care at night, are probably counter-productive in terms of professional development. First, they reinforce the perennial problem among night nurses – a sense of 'apartness'. Secondly, they reinforce the notion that there can be lower expectations of professional nurses working at night than of those who work only by day. Nurses ought to be able to exercise an informed choice between day work and night work, or a combination of the two. In terms of professional development no distinction should be made.

References

Downie R S and Calman K C (1987) *Healthy Respect*. London: Faber and Faber.
Kemp J (1989) *Nursing at Night*. Unpublished MPhil Thesis, University of Hull.
NHS Management Consultancy Services (1987) *Study of Night Nursing Services*. London: DHSS.
Royal College of Nursing (1958) *The Problem of Providing a Continuous Nursing Service Especially in Relation to Night Duty*. London: Royal College of Nursing.
Storey M (1986) Towards the Year 2000. *The Professional Nurse*, May 1986.

Chapter 11
Issues in Nursing
Fiona Wilkinson

I start this chapter by making two assumptions for which I make no apology. Firstly, this book has set out to discuss the special role, responsibilities and needs of night nurses. While the work of night nurses in some respects is different from that of day nurses, their contribution to patient care is no less valuable, and issues which face nursing are relevant to all nurses. By reinforcing this message it is hoped to move further away from the 'them and us' attitude which commonly prevails between day and night nurses. Secondly, in no small part due to successive government initiatives for the management of health, the NHS operates in a changing environment. Thus an author might expect that a discussion of current and future issues in nursing could be superseded before it is even published. This author believes that it is unrealistic to think that current changes in the NHS and their far-reaching implications will be reversed and that consequently this chapter will remain topical.

The New Look NHS

At the end of January 1989, the then Health Secretary Kenneth Clarke announced the results of the NHS review, the White Paper 'Working for Patients'. The review is aimed at making the NHS more business-like by introducing market forces into the service. This is being done by a number of financial and structural changes. These include:

- allowing NHS hospitals to opt out of district control and become self-governing;
- creating an internal market by allowing health authorities to buy care from each other;
- restructuring health authorities;
- allowing GPs to hold their own budgets.

Some have put forward the notion that the hidden agenda behind the government reforms is the wish to divert expensive health care provision away from London. The dilemma for government has been how to achieve this without directly closing some of the large and famous London teaching hospitals. This would be politically damaging in such a Tory stronghold as London and 'Roseland' (i.e. the rest of South East England). However it is likely that the creation of an internal market will force at least one of the London teaching hospitals to close (probably St Thomas'), as it will not be able to attract enough 'business' in the new competitive market environment.

The timing for the changes was April 1991 following the passing of the National Health Service and Community Care Act in June 1990. There has been much criticism of the government concerning the unrealistic timetable for change. Health Service managers all over the country have been striving to meet seemingly impossible deadlines to make major changes. These changes hold both opportunities and dangers for nurses.

Self-Governing Trusts

One of the most controversial proposals in the White Paper has been the establishment of NHS Self-Governing Trusts. Applications for trust status are being received by the Department of Health from all types of hospitals as well as community units, units providing specific types of care (for example mental health), and even complete health districts. As the name implies, these Trusts will be self-governing, in other words fully managing their affairs and not accountable to the district health authority. Each Trust is run by a board of five executive and five non-executive directors. Among the executive directors is a senior nurse, a general manager, a medical director and a finance director. This is unlike the newly restructured health authorities where in some instances there will be no nursing input at the most senior level.

So what are the implications of NHS Trusts for nurses? The most negatively perceived aspect is the issue of pay and conditions. These will no longer be negotiated nationally, but will be up to the directors of the Trust to pay what they wish, and to determine conditions of employment. If this is the case there may be a knock-on effect for nurses working for district health authority controlled hospitals (directly managed units). It is possible that national pay negotiators will have diminished negotiating power because they will no longer be acting for all unionised nurses. However, to date there is evidence that Trusts are maintaining nationally negotiated pay agreements. Inevitably, in the long term, Trusts will use their freedom to pay higher salaries where nurses are in short supply. This is already true in London where some theatre and intensive nurses can secure enhanced salaries.

It is the government's stated aim to dismantle the Whitley negotiating machinery and introduce locally determined pay for all nurses, not just those working for self-governing Trusts. Together with the effect of the shortage of 15 to 25 year olds entering the job market in 1992/93, this may herald an upward spiral in nurses pay.

Any pay benefits must be set in the context of how nurses are going to be employed in the future. The stress on quality within the NHS reforms means that services will have to become more flexible to the needs of patients, for example providing outpatients services outside the traditional hours of 9–5 Monday to Friday. To achieve such changes and to control staff costs and so remain competitive it is likely that hospitals will reduce their numbers of full time (i.e. core) staff across all professional groups and increase their numbers of contract staff. Contract staff are self-employed workers who are attracted to an hourly contract arrangement that may vary according to personal circumstances. The distinction between core and contract staff will enable service providers to work towards a flexibility that allows staffing and labour costs to vary more in proportion with patient flow.

If NHS trusts expand and entrepreneurial ideas are the order of the day, there is an opportunity for nurses to make major contributions to new thinking at local level and to have a clear leadership role. Of course, this is dependent on nurses coming to terms with and grasping the opportunities which the internal market will bring.

The Internal Market

The White Paper has signalled the end of the elaborate RAWP (Resource Allocation Working Party) formula of distributing money to health authorities. Regional health authorities will be funded according to population, weighted to reflect health and age distribution and the relative costs of providing services. In turn, in allocating funds to districts, regions will be taking into consideration the resident populations of their districts.

Under the NHS reforms districts have taken on a role of both purchasers of services and providers of services. In their purchasing role they are endeavouring to buy the best services they can from their own hospitals, other district health authority hospitals, Self-Governing Trusts or the private sector, and in the future from local authorities. In their provider role districts are specifying the services their units provide and are free to offer their services to different districts.

The implications for nurses in this new scenario of purchasers and providers mainly fall within the associated revised management arrangements. To set the most recent changes into context it is necessary to go back seven years to the publication of the Griffiths management report in 1983 which brought us general management. Figure 11.1 illustrates the organisational structure of most district health authorities between 1984 and 1990. During this period only a handful of senior nurses were appointed to general management posts at regional, district and local level.

Robinson (1989), in a four year study into the progress of Britain's top nurses in the post-Griffiths NHS, concluded that nursing at this time was in a state of little coherence and, very often, in depressing confusion. In many district health authorities the chief nurse role had been diverted into general management with the loss of pure nursing advice at district level.

The purchaser/provider split has resulted in a large organisational change at district level. We are now seeing the amalgamation of some smaller district purchasers into consortia so increasing their purchasing power. As yet few people from the nursing ranks are in senior purchasing authority roles. Under this restructuring each regional and district health authority now has five executive and five non-executive members with no mandate for the inclusion of a nurse member. So it seems that at a strategic planning level the rug is being further pulled from under nurses in the way they are able to influence

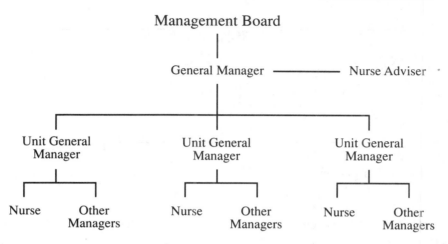

Figure 11.1 Organisational Structure 1984–1990

the future of the NHS. This uneasy relationship with NHS management is further strained by the emergence of clinical directorates.

Clinical Directorates

This is the term given to a clinical management model which involves doctors in the management of clinical services. For those nurses who have been arguing that leadership should come from those more closely involved with clinical practice, the post of a clinical director with the responsibility of a budget, seems tailor made for a nurse. However this does not achieve the political objective of controlling consultants who spend the largest proportion of NHS resources. Therefore the overwhelming majority of these jobs are going to doctors, although many are resisting the pressures to take on the new responsibility of budget holding which they see as a method of controlling any extravagant misuse of clinical freedom.

Within these new organisational arrangements, nurses at operational level are accountable to a manager at directorate level (usually but not always a nurse), with the nursing post at unit level either being dispensed with or acting as an adviser to the unit general manager. Figure 11.2 illustrates one clinical management model. This model is highly decentralised with the consultant clinical director coordinating consultant colleagues and managing clinical services staff.

Where directorates have been introduced, the majority of these new structures are in their infancy. However, there is already clear evidence that in some areas rather than assisting to develop a corporate culture within a provider unit, such structures are divisive. There are examples of nurses within directorates refusing to lend equipment and supplies to other directorates and 'shielding' empty beds in order to protect tight budgets. So it continues to be a very difficult time for senior nurses and every nurse, at whatever level of the service he or she is working at, should be concerned.

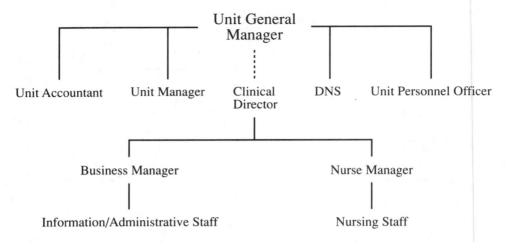

Figure 11.2 Clinical managerment model

The changes in management structures are happening now but will affect the working environment of clinical nurses tomorrow. This is particularly true within the community care part of the new NHS Act.

Caring For People

The community care part of the new NHS and Community Care Act was presented as a government White Paper, 'Caring for People', shortly after the White Paper 'Working for Patients'. 'Caring for People' radically alters community care for elderly, mentally ill, mentally handicapped and disabled people. Under the new plan local authorities will be providing social care and health authorities providing health care, areas which may seem difficult to separate.

Health authorities are purchasers of health care for their resident populations and will only wish to purchase services (such as community nurses) that are truly for health. Managers of community health services will quickly need to start determining what service they are providing. They will have to attempt to separate health from social care. They will have to be explicit about the criteria they use for admitting and discharging patients into the care of community nursing staff, and they will have to ensure the development of quality measuring tools that will demonstrate the effectiveness of the service being provided.

The survival of the district nursing and health visiting service will be dependent on GPs and health authorities wishing to purchase those services. However, some GPs may choose to employ their own staff to provide the services required by their practice population rather than contract with health authorities or community units for the provision of those services. This is likely in the light of the new GP contract which rewards GPs who provide a comprehensive service to their elderly patients which includes carrying out health assessments. GPs may wish to employ their own district nurses and health visitors to undertake this work on their behalf. Community units as we know them today may cease to be viable entities. However, although the management structure under which community nurses currently operate may change, the skills they offer will be in greater demand than ever before. In future local authorities will be responsible for case management and for arranging key workers to ensure patient needs are met. It is unlikely that social workers will have the skills and expertise associated with these tasks, at least in the short term. It is to their community nursing colleagues that they will look for help and support in carrying out their new responsibilities.

We are likely to witness the emergence of a variety of models of management for community nursing provision. Groups of nurses setting up their own agencies and contracting their services to GPs and health authorities could become the norm. In the new order of things community nurses may, for the first time, be able to use the skills and knowledge they acquired in nurse education establishments.

Nurse Education

One of the major policies which will reshape nursing is most certainly Project 2000 (1986). With many programmes now well under way the effect the new curricula will have on the development of the clinical role of nursing is an issue which requires close scrutiny.

What does the new curriculum contain? While it is recognised that the applied biological sciences are still essential, more emphasis is now being placed on social sciences, such as health psychology and ethics. Ethics is an especially vital component. Pashley (1989) concludes that ethics is not only vital for nurses in their everyday practice, but also for educators who, perhaps for the first time, need an understanding of educational ethics as they encourage their students to question the way in which care is provided. Another element of the new curriculum is research, with an emphasis on bridging the theory/practice gap and ensuring research underpins clinical practice.

One of the fundamental issues in nurse education is whether Project 2000 will enhance the clinical role of the nurse or will the qualified clinical nurse disappear and more reliance be placed on the health care assistant? Of course there is no definitive answer to this question, but the two sides of the debate are presented here.

At present, it costs about £17 000 to train each student nurse, but a health authority recoups around £14 000 of this by way of the student's service input while training. With Project 2000 there is less service input (but not less clinical experience than at present) and therefore it begs the question will health authorities wish to put money into education without receiving the service input? Health authorities might find short-term costs exceeding the long-term benefits and invest instead in the service based health care assistant. This is of particular concern to night nurses where there are traditionally a greater number of nursing auxiliaries. Where do they fit into the new scheme of things? Nurses are concerned that they will become the supervisors of this unqualified group of workers who will take on clinical nursing duties and fill the gaps left by the new supernumerary nurse students.

In support of the argument that Project 2000 will enhance the clinical role of the nurse are the proposed plans for postbasic education. The aim is to develop a systematic review of clinical practice and in this way maintain standards of clinical practice. The UKCC is responsible for standards of training and conduct of the profession, but currently have no formal method of acknowledging continuing education and therefore no way of knowing if standards are being maintained. Of course this makes the assumption that prevailing standards are worthy of maintenance. The new proposals put forward by the UKCC are known as the Post-Registration Education and Practice Project (PREPP).

The PREPP team have identified three levels at which practitioners can develop. These are: practice following initial registration; specialist practice; and advanced practice. Many nurses will remain in the first level all their working lives, gaining experience and educational qualifications throughout, which help them improve the way they work.

A specialist practitioner will be someone who has, following initial registration, undertaken specific education in a clearly defined specialty such as intensive care nursing. Advanced practice will be more concerned with pioneering and developing new roles and areas of practice, through research, education or clinical innovation. The proposals within PREPP raise several issues worth mentioning:

- The measure of professional competence seems to be focused on formal study, which for night nurses is often particularly difficult to achieve. Could not the UKCC develop a way of acknowledging professional advancement through practice and experience?
- The PREPP initiative requires the right administrative system with the people to operate it and the money to implement it. Who is going to assess the individual nurse's personal development? It could be done by peer review or as part of the more traditional individual performance review.
- The ultimate measure of PREPP's value must be its impact on patient care.

A second point in support of Project 2000 enhancing the clinical role of the nurse is that Project 2000 curricula are being implemented by teams of nurse educators, higher education sector educators and with greater involvement of nurse practitioners themselves. Thirdly, there is a great deal of encouragement being given for the recruitment of the mature student into the profession, and most of these people are keen to work in clinical practice and stay there. Fourthly, the proposed widening of the entry gate into nursing will provide for the gradual progression of health care assistants who are willing and able to enter nursing programmes. Last but by no means least, there is the development of an approach to nursing, the success of which is dependent on the availability of skilled clinical practitioners. This approach is primary nursing.

Primary Nursing

Primary nursing is a concept which focuses on the idea of 'partnership' between nurses and patients and 'accountability'. It is a concept which is not new and already operates throughout the world (Otaya 1979, Medaglia 1978). The popularity of primary nursing is increasing among nurses in this country.

Following a nursing assessment a patient is allocated to a primary nurse who plans the care with that patient and is accountable for the care received for the duration the patient receives care. The primary nurse is supported by associate nurses who carry out the prescribed care with, and in the absence of, the primary nurse.

Primary nursing requires the redefinition of individual nurses' roles and responsibilities. For example the night sister will become a supporter, educator and clinical specialist, but will no longer be directly accountable for nursing care delivered at night. Within a hospital setting the staff nurse will act as ward co-ordinator and will be an associate nurse, along with enrolled nurses, auxiliaries and learners.

Most of the literature on primary nursing designates night staff as associate nurses. Day staff have greater opportunity to contact other members of the multi-disciplinary team, so they usually become the primary nurses.

Care planning done by night staff for night time admissions is usually confined to immediate care only. Excepting unforeseen circumstances occurring at night, the primary nurse will prescribe the care to be given at night. In reality this may already happen in your existing care system, the difference with primary nursing is that night staff will be accountable to the primary nurse on day duty, and ultimately to the day ward sister for the care they give. Qualified night staff may feel adversely affected by the introduction of primary nursing. For instance, newly qualified staff nurses may feel that their care prescribing role can be fully realised only as primary nurses, which means they must switch to day shifts. More experienced night staff may find it difficult to accept care prescribed by less experienced day primary nurses.

So as you can see, primary nursing has far-reaching consequences for permanent night staff, not least on the issue of accountability and autonomy.

Accountability and Autonomy in Nursing Practice

Accountability can be described as the formal obligation to disclose what you have done. Once you have accepted responsibility for any given task you can be held to account. Put into the context of nursing this means that through accepting your registration you can be held accountable by the UKCC for your professional actions; by accepting and carrying out a job you can be held to account by your employing authority; and by carrying out clinical care you can be held to account by your patient. If nurses are to be accountable for the care they provide, there is a fundamental issue to be addressed, particularly for night nurses – it is the manner in which the work is organised. If night staff have a different allocation of patients on a night-to-night basis, as seems to happen so often, it is questionable that they can get to know patients well enough to be held to account.

Autonomy can be considered to be the power or right to self-govern. There is a fine line between the freedom to practise autonomously and total freedom of action, the latter being unacceptable professional practice. Perhaps it is more appropriate to be working towards cohesion and teamwork. The whole question of accountability and autonomy raises the issue that unless nurses are sure what it is they do, they are not in a position to fulfil leadership roles or to be accountable. Neither do they have the right to seek acceptance as autonomous practitioners. Nurses must face the fact that there is considerable confusion about just what it is they can or cannot do and must consider what they are seeking. There is a path to be chosen.

So what are the options open to nursing? Two paths which have been identified are those of extension and expansion (McFarlane 1980, Pearson 1983, Orlando 1987). In this context extension means the acceptance of new tasks, frequently delegated from other occupational groups, in particular medicine, and often related to the acquisition of specific technical skills. Obvious examples are the performance of venepuncture and ECGs. Expansion of nursing is a totally different concept. This recognises the true value of nursing as a separate therapeutic activity in its own right, helping patients to reach predefined health related goals which may or may not be associated with the cure of disease. Expansion does not necessarily exclude extension. With expansion, the decision as to which skills should be learnt is based on each practitioner's particular situation, rather than being delegated from outside the profession, as the extended role may be. For years now nursing has been moving down a road of extension, and for Orlando (1987), this raises significant fears. The major issue she sees is that extension leads to dependence. It can be argued that if such a path is followed, nurses will perpetuate the monopoly over resources and access to treatment which is held by the medical profession. It seems that if the extended path alone is followed, there is a risk that the caring component of nursing may be lost in the rush to gain new technical skills. Vaughan (1989) argues that nursing has already lost some of its unique functions. She states that 'over a period of years, nurses have allowed their role to become eroded by passing on social welfare to social workers, body movement to physiotherapists and activities to occupational therapists, all of which have their origins in nursing.'

If nurses continue to extend into delegated technical functions with a consequent splitting off of fragments of care, then what used to be known as nursing will be lost for ever. This does not in any way devalue the contribution that specialists or occupational groups make to health care, but it does challenge the way in which nurses work with them and the use of nursing skills.

Nursing Skills

An area of clinical practice that is currently under scrutiny is the tasks that nurses are carrying out and the skills needed to perform them. Although the debate surrounding skill mix is not new (a major DHSS review took place in 1986), the drive for providing a cost-efficient and effective service has meant it is again at the top of the agenda for many senior nurses. Another reason for the renewed interest in activity and skill mix is connected with clinical regrading. It is generally accepted that clinical regrading has been implemented in an inconsistent and poorly managed way. The debate has been most vociferous among night nurses with many sisters graded lower than their day counterparts who are designated as having continuing responsibility of care.

It is probable that the regrading exercise has heralded the start of major reprofiling work. There is a long established pattern of demarcation between professionally, technically and commercially qualified groups of staff. For example, doctor and nurse, technician and pathologist, radiographer and radiologist etc. Reprofiling is about altering the demarcation boundaries in order to optimise the utilisation of staff to increase efficiency and effectiveness and so enabling more patients to be treated without compromising quality.

Early in 1989 a call for a review of nursing tasks and procedures came from the chief nursing officer for England, in the form of a letter to all regional and district nursing officers telling them that nurses must relinquish many unnecessary routine tasks which they have traditionally performed. Not surprisingly this received a mixed response from the profession. The early response of both the Royal College of Nursing and the UKCC was to express concern at the contents of the letter. Some nurses have taken a more positive view and see that by taking a fresh look at the type of nursing interventions, the quality of service can be improved. This seems to be part of a drive to devolve more responsibility to clinical nurses for the service they provide. One way of facilitating this process has been to involve clinical nurses in resource management.

Resource Management

Resource management was introduced by the NHS Management Board in 1986. Its aim, the board said, was to: 'enable the NHS to give a better service to its patients by helping clinical staff and other managers to make more informed judgement about how the resources they control can be used to maximum effect'. The idea of helping health authorities improve the use of their resources is nothing new, but the difference this time is the availability of information on which to make those decisions. The information about the resources available for patient care, in other words people, time and equipment, will be produced on a much more scientific basis than before.

Initially there were six resource management pilot sites. The project was extended to fifty sites during 1989/90 and further development of the project is planned. Each unit has evolved its own approach to resource management. Some have concentrated on involving doctors and nurses in the management process by creating clinical directorates, referred to earlier in this chapter. The directorates have responsibility for how money is spent and how future spending is planned in their unit.

So, in the future what will resource management mean for nurses at the sharp end of care? There will be an increased awareness of costs of everyday items and accountability for budgets will mean that nurses will be more careful about lending. It is likely that wards and units will 'charge' other sections of their organisation for borrowing equipment and staff. This could be to the benefit of patients as shortfalls in the service will not be hidden. However carefully staff at clinical level control budgets, problems will arise if overall funding for a unit is reduced.

Resource management is impossible to implement without technology to provide and process the necessary information. To date most nurses manage in a structure which provides them with very little information. The only information most ward sisters receive is when the unit is overspent and they are told to cut back. They have nothing to tell them why, or how to remedy the situation. So the success of resource management is dependent on information technology.

Information Technology

Resource management involves providing detailed information on each patient, including diagnosis, procedures and therapeutic events. In this way patient profiles can be reviewed with other patients of a similar type and the use of resources compared – case mix management. Nursing information systems will be important feeder systems to case mix management systems as the use of nursing skills is a major resource, comprising about 40 per cent of an acute hospital budget. Nursing information systems have been in development since the 1960s. However these developments focused on discrete and specific areas such as nurse tracking (personnel), learner allocation and latterly rostering and care planning. The result has been a number of systems which address some areas but not all, leading to multiple systems purchase which are difficult to interface. The potential benefit in terms of saving nurse time was unrealised with these systems. The most recent nurse management systems enable the systematic collection of a variety of nurse and patient data to ensure the most effective and efficient use of the nursing resource. Figure 11.3 shows some of the information interchanges which will be facilitated by computer technology.

Information use must support the philosophy of nursing to ensure the emphasis on cost and efficiency does not detract from providing individualised patient care. Nurses will be required to become computer literate to enable them not only to use computer systems but to design, develop and evaluate nursing systems. These are skills which have not generally been uppermost in the minds of women in nursing.

Women in Nursing

In 1989 a report from the National Steering Group on Equal Opportunities for Women in the NHS showed that women working in the health service, many of them in nursing, receive a poor deal. The lack of work-break

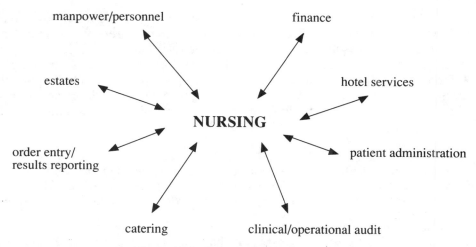

Figure 11.3 Information interchanges

schemes, flexible working hours, demotion if returning on a part-time basis and lack of childcare facilities are the main issues. The report gathers together some sound ideas about work-break schemes, job sharing, providing continuing education for part-time workers and reviewing selection procedures. The suggestions are nothing new but the introduction of equal opportunities has remained scattered and unco-ordinated. However, there may be some hope on the horizon due to the increasing shortage of staff and gloomy prospects for recruitment for many health authorities. This situation presents a golden opportunity for nurses to push for change. It is an opportunity which must not be missed.

The Implications of the European Economic Community Changes in 1992

In 1957 six countries (Belgium, France, Germany, Netherlands, Italy and Luxembourg) signed the Treaty of Rome and set up the European Economic Community and a European Atomic Energy Community. There are now twelve members (including Britain), and the debate over the entry of a thirteenth – Turkey – is hotting up. The Single European Act, which came into effect in July 1987, 'reinforced the commitment to create a single unified market in which the free movement of goods, persons, services and capital is assured' (Croner 1989). In 1992, the remaining barriers to trade were removed.

The European Community also pursues social and environmental goals. Much work has been done on the setting of standards of goods, standards of health and safety in the workplace, and training within key professions. Directives relating to general nurse training have been in place since 1979, and for midwifery since 1983. They ensure that any nurse or midwife from a member state who completed their training after 1979 and 1983 respectively is entitled to registration in any other member state. Nurses who qualified before these dates require a certificate that states they have been 'effectively and lawfully' engaged in general nursing for at least three out of five years prior to their application to work in another member state. Still under discussion are directives relating to psychiatric and paediatric nurse training.

Of course, being able to register in a country does not mean you will necessarily get a job. Usually the greatest obstacle is the language barrier and it will be up to the individual nurse to improve his or her linguistic skills.

References

Croner's Europe (1989) Kingston upon Thames: Croner Publications Ltd.

DHSS (1986) *Mix and Match: A Review of Nursing Skill Mix*. London: DHSS.

DHSS (1988) *The National Health Service Management Inquiry (Griffiths Report)*. London: DHSS.

McFarlane J (1980) *Essays on Nursing*. London: Kings Fund.

Medaglia M (1978) A coronary care unit implements primary nursing. *Canadian Nurse*, **74**, 32–34.

National Steering Group on Equal Opportunities for Women in the NHS (1989) *Equal Opportunities for Women in the NHS*.

Orlando J (1987) Nursing in the 21st century – alternative paths. *Journal of Advanced Nursing*, **12**, 4, 405–412.

Otoya T (1979) Advantages and disadvantages of team nursing: a trial of primary nursing. *Kangogaku Zasshi*, **43**, 163–169.

Pashley G (1989) *Report on the Curriculum for RMN: Need for Research*, paper given at Lancaster University Centre for Health Research.

Pearson A (1983) *The Clinical Nursing Unit*. London: Heinemann.

Robinson J, Strong P and Elkan R (1989) *Griffiths and the Nurses: A National Survey of CNAs*. University of Warwick: Nursing Policy Studies Centre.

United Kingdom Central Council (1986) *Project 2000: A New Preparation for Practice*. London: UKCC.

Vaughan B (1989) Autonomy and accountability. *Nursing Times*, January 18, **85**, 3.

Chapter 12
The Way Forward
Richard McMahon

Introduction

Nursing is developing rapidly and radically. Not only is clinical knowledge advancing, but also the way nursing is managed is changing, so that account-ability is clearer and problems are more quickly identified and solved. The care of patients at night is being swept along in this tide of change. In the first chapter, six problems for nursing were identified as needing to be challenged if a quality night service is to be achieved. In this chapter, those issues will be addressed, and a variety of responses will be offered.

The care of patients at night cannot be ignored in the hospital service, not least because under the 'new' National Health Service that came into being on April 1st 1991, Health Authorities have service contracts with the providers of care, meaning hospitals and other organisations. Those service contracts have three elements: the quality of care, the quantity of care and the cost of care. Nurses must ensure that they are providing a quality service on a 24 hour a day basis. At the same time, rest and sleep are essential for health and healing (Canavan 1986, Torrance 1990) and a return to independence for a patient means being able to cope at night as well as during the day. Providing a high quality caring service at night may have a significant effect on the quantity of patients a hospital treats in a year. Finally, the cost of care is under close scrutiny. The grades and skill-mix of staff on duty must be justified if it is not to be radically altered in an effort to keep costs to a minimum. The need to develop the care of patients at night, and the night nursing service as a whole, has never been more urgent.

The Challenges to Nursing

In Chapter 1 the following issues were identified as needing to be addressed by nurses:

- lack of research into clinical problems at night;
- maximising performance of nurses working at night;
- nurses at night becoming pro-active and therapeutic in their care;
- bridging the divide between day and night staff;

- redressing the imbalance in training and other facilities available for nurses working at night;
- retaining expertise and a career structure for night nurses.

These will now be examined individually.

Lack of Research

The amount of research into care at night is increasing slowly, with the Department of Health indicating the importance of this area by commissioning three further studies into the subject. However, much of the focus has been on organisational rather than clinical issues. In many ways this reflects the pattern of much of the early nursing research, however many nurses now have the skills to examine clinical issues. Much exploratory work has already been done, for example in relation to night-time drinks. Morgan et al (1989) found that a significant number of elderly insomniacs also drink tea at night. Whilst the effect of caffeine in disturbing sleep has been well documented (Karacan et al 1976, Levy and Zylber-Katz 1983), for some people making tea is also a response to sleeplessness. It is common practice for nurses to offer tea to wakeful patients in the middle of the night, however the efficacy of this practice has not been tested, particularly in relation to whether the individual is accustomed to drinking tea at that time at home. It may be that for anxious patients in hospital the desire for a cup of tea, and the human contact that comes with it, may outweigh the desire to go to sleep. Suppositions such as these are worthy of investigation by nurses, and many other questions arise out research done into the actual and potential effects of other bedtime drinks such as milk beverages (Brezinova and Oswald 1972, Adam 1980), alcohol (Rundell et al 1972) and carbonated soft drinks (Darragh et al 1979).

Clearly the need and potential for research into clinical issues at night is immense, and there is no reason why a greater number of nurses who commonly work at night cannot develop the skills and knowledge necessary to start to find answers to these questions for themselves.

Maximising Performance

Helping nurses who work the night shift either permanently or on rotation to feel well in themselves is a major challenge which can directly influence the quality of care. Night shift workers frequently suffer from gastro-intestinal disorders, headaches, tiredness and irritability (Armstrong 1987), due to the disruption of their circadian rhythms. Nurses experiencing any of these symptoms whilst they are on duty may have their potential to give good care compromised as well as the personal stress that suffering such effects on a regular basis must cause. Recommendations for shift patterns which 'advance' the body clock (Minors et al 1985) for nurses who work internal rotation have not been implemented in all hospitals. Similarly, it has to be acknowledged that many nurses who work regular nights are doubly disadvantaged in that they not only work in the hours of darkness, but also have great social responsibilities at home. Minors et al (1985) recommend that blocks of nights should last three or four nights; this should only be extended where the individual has the social circumstances and motivation to become 'nocturnal', and shortened where the nurse can have several days off to adjust.

Apart from 'user friendly' shift systems, hospitals have a responsibility to provide support in other ways. Lloyd (1989) suggests that Occupational Health Departments should take an interest in the health problems of night workers, not least by occasionally being available at a time when they can offer health assessment and advice to these workers. In view of the gastro-intestinal disorders experienced by night workers, hospitals should provide a quality meals service at night, which if it cannot be manned, is set up in such a way that it cannot be accessed by the staff or public before night duty starts.

The Need to Become Therapeutic and Proactive in Practice

Nursing as a whole has often been described as a 'caretaking' activity (Evers 1981a and b) whilst other health workers 'heal' the patient; within nursing itself many nurses have viewed the work of their night shift colleagues as 'babysitting'. In Chapter 1 the need for more nurses to recognise that a patient's day and night-time functioning are interdependent was identified. If nurses are to give care which maximises the patient's potential, then they must take a genuinely holistic approach.

Being proactive in care often involves addressing many issues in the management of care. For example it has been suggested (McMahon 1990) that medical interventions such as non-emergency blood transfusions occur at night for the convenience of the nurses, rather than with regard to the needs of the patient who may suffer sleep deprivation as a result of the regularity of the observations being performed.

Therapeutic nursing is nursing which deliberately achieves beneficial outcome with patients. McMahon (1991) identified six therapeutic activities in nursing:

1. Developing partnership, intimacy and reciprocity in the nurse-patient relationship;
2. manipulating the environment;
3. teaching;
4. providing comfort;
5. adopting complementary health practices; and
6. utilising tested physical interventions.

Nurses who work at night must themselves take up the challenge of developing their practice to fulfil these activities.

1. Communicating effectively with patients involves nurses in having a repertoire of skills from which they can choose appropriately for the individual they are with. Indeed, tentative interpretation of research data (Ersser 1991) seems to support the view that being with the patient in

an open, wholehearted and available way is perceived as being therapeutic by patients (Paterson and Zderad 1976).

2. There is much evidence that environmental factors have a major influence
on patients' satisfaction with their care at night (Ogilvie 1980, Closs
1988), and nurses must be proactive in setting standards for noise, light,
temperature and other variables during the hours of darkness.

3. Therapeutic nurses at night must adopt teaching as a fundamental part
of their role. In relation to sleep, the effective nurse should, where
appropriate, be informing the patient about the effects of such activities
as smoking on sleeplessness (Soldatos et al 1980) and teaching the anxious
patient relaxation techniques (see Morgan 1987, pp 126–130). Also, if
nursing is to provide a uniform service, then the nurse working the night
shift must be as capable as the nurses on any other shift to maintain a
patient's education programme for teaching him about managing his own
colostomy, lifting himself up the bed or whatever his needs are.

4. Comfort is a necessity for promoting sleep. Intervening to relieve and
prevent the recurrence of pain has been identified as a major issue (see
Chapter 6). Other nursing actions can make a major difference to the
patient trying to sleep; his own pillow from home, careful positioning,
relief of a full bladder should all be considered and acted upon by the
therapeutic nurse at night.

5. Complementary health practices have much to offer at night, e.g. the use
of essential oils to create a pleasant environment, massage to create
relaxation. Nurses who care at night may well have the space in their
working hours to spend time administering complementary therapies.
Such nurses must take the initiative in ensuring that they have the necessary training and experience to perform these therapies.

6. Many aspects of care now have research evidence to help the nurse decide
the most appropriate interventions. Continued reliance on outdated and
discredited practices is incompatible with therapeutic nursing, and it is
the responsibility of all nurses to implement sound relevant research in
their practice.

If these ideas are put together, the idea of 'actively settling' patients at the
beginning of the night emerges as the type of practice a therapeutic night
nurse might adopt. This practice addresses the issue of night nursing being a
'reactive and demand led service' (NHS Management Consultancy Services
1987), and may be simply described as follows. Instead of a nurse flitting
from one patient to the next in response to patients calling, once immediate
needs are dealt with the nurse should reassure each patient being cared for
that they will be settled for the night. The nurse can then spend quality time
with patients, taking steps to maximise their comfort, anticipate problems
and plan care for the rest of the night. By the way nurses communicate with
patients they can convince them that they genuinely want them to call if they
need a nurse.

The Day/Night Divide

One of the most entrenched attitudes to be found on hospital wards is the 'them and us' phenomenon between night and day staff. It is almost expected that each shift should blame the other for breakdowns in care or communication. Stories abound of night nurses tucking themselves up to sleep for the rest of the shift after cocooning incontinent patients in enough pads to see them through the night. Even where the night staff are not considered to be guilty of anything more than spending the night knitting, the work of the night nurse is often seen as being less valuable. From the perspective of the night nurse, many factors have led to, and perpetuated this day/night divide.

- Lack of contact between the two groups. The nurses from each group rarely work or meet socially with each other, leading them to make assumptions about those who work the opposite shift.
- The social circumstances which make many nurses choose night duty militate against them when it comes to attending courses or participating in training. Also, many people who return to nursing after a significant break restart work on nights without updating.
- For many years there has been a strict division of labour between night and day-time workers. This allocation of jobs has frequently led to resentment when one or other group has been unable to complete its allotted tasks before the end of the shift.
- In many areas weak nurse management placed problem workers on night duty and failed to support nurses already on that shift who were not coping. Along with this the skill-mix on nights has often been heavily weighted towards the employment of untrained staff. Together these factors have meant that often the quality of individuals working at night has not been the same as on days. It is easy to imagine how this can create a self-perpetuating problem whereby 'good' nurses are reluctant to join or stay with a team which lacks ability, enthusiasm or potential.
- Many nurses who care at night do not themselves recognise or demonstrate the specialist aspects of much of their work.

It is up to nurses to bridge the day/night divide so that day and night staff work as colleagues rather than as rivals. This involves changing attitudes and implementing radical solutions. Firstly, ward teams must recognise that the division into day and night work is a false one, as patients' needs are not related to shift times. The potential quality of care should be uniform throughout the day and night, and nurses should be explicit in their considering each individual patient in terms of his 24-hour functioning.

Perhaps most critically for the nurses who work at night, they feel that their work should be valued. It should be recognised that in the vast majority of cases where nurses have not been active all night it is not because they have been 'lazy' or chosen an easy option, rather the quietness of the night is as a direct result of excellent nursing care in helping a large group of patients to sleep all night.

The DHSS report (NHS Management Consultancy Services 1987) observed that separate night and day staff perpetuated the 'them and us'. Many wards have moved to internal rotation with the aim of creating a unified staff. Whilst this can rarely be achieved quickly, it may be gradually introduced and extended as vacancies arise. However, if the concept of a unified nursing team is a serious goal, it is worth considering abandoning the terminology of 'day staff' or 'day nurses' and 'night staff' or 'night nurses'. Such semantics may seem trivial; however the abandonment of the term 'geriatrics' by all disciplines except medicine and the media has made a significant statement about the way we view elderly people.

The lack of professional and social contact between the groups of staff can be eased by occasional 'job swaps' between nurses, or by ensuring that ward meetings take place at a time when the largest number of staff representing different groups can attend. It may be that nurses who work predominantly at night will have to demand that meetings are held at a time when they can easily attend. Once there they must contribute in a positive and enthusiastic way. Similarly, the practice of having separate social events for nurses who work in the day and those who work at night is divisive. As with all issues, the ward staff should be viewed by all as a unified group.

Finally, the problem of nurses with limited abilities being sent or selecting themselves on to nights needs to be addressed. Training must be available for nurses who predominantly work unsocial hours to update themselves. If the recommendations of the Post Registration Education and Practice Project (PREPP) (1990) are implemented, nurses who have been out of practice for five or more years will have to complete a return to practice course. The setting of standards and the use of objective setting through individual performance review are steps towards identifying nurses who are not performing to an adequate standard. However, in future nurse managers should confront problems among staff rather than simply transfer miscreants to night duty.

Redressing the Imbalance in Training and Other Facilities

Whilst the PREPP Report provides ammunition for nurses who care at night to demand training, the minimum amount of five days every three years is probably inadequate for the needs of most nurses. Nurses who work at night need to identify their learning needs and how these may be met as a group and as individuals.

A good example of how nurses who work mainly at night can help themselves is provided by 'Sobell House', the hospice at the Churchill Hospital in Oxford, where the nurses have set up a night duty group with the following aims:

- to meet the continuing education needs of night staff;
- to provide informal support;
- to provide a way in which night staff can become involved in ward developments and discussions.

The group meets once per month, often with a speaker chosen by the group attending. The meetings take place at 8pm and a different weekday night is chosen for each session to allow as many people as possible to attend. Such initiatives have the advantage of the control and power within the group lying with the practitioners themselves.

It is also useful on a hospital or unit-wide basis for nurses who work predominantly at night to unite to call for training opportunities, facilities and educational support. Clearly an active group which can work politically can achieve far more than a few enthusiastic, but isolated, individuals. Such a unified group may not only create change in the provision of learning opportunities, but also in other aspects of night work identified in Chapter 1, such as security needs.

Retaining Expertise and a Career Structure

It is fairly certain that clinging to old management structures and practices at night will lead to a continued erosion of grading and status of night nurses. However, that is not to say that there is no longer a need for higher grade nurses at night, rather that new and innovative roles which better meet the needs of the patients and the organisation must be developed. For example, night managers must make their role in monitoring and improving quality an explicit one.

A different approach would be to achieve continuing education at night by developing a clinical practice development role to work with nurses in groups and with individuals. The post would be an attractive one as it would still be based in practice, but would also have teaching and change-facilitating aspects. Such a person could work with individuals of all grades, as well as holding short teaching sessions in the night for nurses from one or more wards.

Another post with enormous potential would be to have a clinical nurse specialist (CNS) in sleep and patient's problems at night. A CNS is a nurse who through study and practice has become an expert in a defined area of clinical nursing. Hamric and Spross (1989) identify four principal roles for a CNS, all of which would be appropriate for one specialising in sleep and other night-time problems.

Expert Practice.   Practice is the fundamental part of the role, assessing individual patients with sleep disorders either since admission or with more long-standing problems. The CNS would be able to offer a host of interventions such as massage, relaxation, behavioural therapies, teaching regarding diet and so on. In liaison with the occupational health department the CNS could also offer advice and treatment ot members of staff who work shifts and who are having sleep related difficulties.

Consultation.   This could be both intra-professional and inter-professional. This would include advising ward nurses on patients she was not treating herself, assessing the night environment on wards, and responding to enquiries on relevant topics. The CNS would also be available for consultation from doctors, GPs, health visitors etc.

Teaching.   This would include both formal and informal teaching of ward nurses as well as teaching nurse learners. In the past, and still to some extent today, students of nursing did not learn about sleep and other night related issues. The CNS could teach them both in the school and in the clinical areas.

Research.   As has been highlighted earlier, there is a very great need to examine further nursing issues as they relate to care at night. For example, nurses consistently overestimate how much sleep their patients have had during the night (Weiss et al 1973, Aurell and Elmqvist 1985), whilst insomniacs underestimate time spent asleep (Carskadon 1976); clearly an investigation into the effects of improved understanding and assessment of patients' sleep by nurses would be useful. A clinical nurse specialist would be well placed to perform such research.

It is important in defining and monitoring the role of the CNS that it meets the needs of the clients, the organisation, and the individual in post, and that those needs are prioritised (Smith 1990). Whilst initially few nurses might be qualified for such a role, as an understanding of the complexities of caring at night become more widely recognised, the opportunities for nurses to obtain those skills will become available.

Creating Change

If nurses who work at night are to be effective in creating a new order, they must become knowledgeable about creating change. A detailed description of how change might be achieved in nursing is beyond the scope of this chapter, and has been the subject of entire books (e.g. Wright 1989), however a brief description of the change process will give a feel for how change can be approached.

   As with many activities which nurses engage in, there are a recognised series of steps which have been identified to improve the likelihood of success. The steps of the change process are:

1.   recognising exactly what the problem is, and identifying all the factors which surround that problem;
2.   assessing the motivation for change amongst colleagues, their ability to take new ideas and practices on board, and the resources (in terms of money, facilities and people) available to support the change;
3.   the person planning the change assessing his or her own motivation and personal resources for the change;
4.   identifying exactly what it is that is to be achieved by the change;
5.   planning exactly what will be done to create the change, and identifying short-term objectives;
6.   implementing the plan, and supporting the change as it comes into effect;
7.   ensuring that the change continues and setting up mechanisms so that it is not reliant on the person who has instigated the change;
8.   evaluating the results of the change to see if the original objective has been met, and considering any unexpected effects of the change.

9. if the change has been implemented successfully, then the person who created the change should be able to turn his or her attention elsewhere without the organisation returning to pre-change practices.

All change should be necessary, planned and introduced sensitively. Change which is imposed by force is rarely effective, and can only be achieved by those with authority. Alternatively, if the person promoting change helps her workmates recognise the need for change and assists them to develop their own solutions, then the change seems to be more effective and lasting. In planning the change, it is often useful to identify key people who influence the opinions of others. By targeting these individuals and working through any resistance which they may have to change, a considerable amount of time and effort may be saved.

Conclusion

The principal purpose of this book has been to improve the quality of care for patients at night. It has been suggested that the division into 'day' and 'night' nursing is a false one and that although patients at night have special needs, nursing should be providing a unified service which has genuinely adopted a holistic approach to care. All nurses who care for patients need an understanding of the inter-dependence of day and night-time functioning. Nurses who regularly or occasionally care for patients during the hours of darkness need to be able to assess patients with particular reference to their care at night. The nurse needs an understanding of the physiology and psychology of sleep if she is to be able to plan and implement therapeutic care on the basis of that assessment. Despite the continued reliance on sleep-inducing drugs by many doctors (see Oswald 1986 and Glover 1986), nurses now know that they have many interventions to offer patients before resorting to hypnotics with their many undesired effects (Gournay 1988, Pawlicki 1985), however research (Halfens et al 1988) indicates that many nurses still work to a medical model when it comes to sleep medication. Nurses who care at night need to be skilled in aspects of care such as pain relief and the use of interpersonal skills if they are to be effective in promoting not only sleep, but also healing in their patients.

As well as the clinical aspects of providing care, there are a number of organisational issues which affect the provision of a nursing service at night. The effects of shift-work in nurses' circadian rhythms, and hence their performance, is a major factor in the management of the service. Similarly, the whole ethos of the NHS is changing rapidly, with a greater emphasis on quality and the cost of services. Nurses who work at night need to have educational opportunities if they are to fulfil their potential for providing excellent care.

Finally, it has been demonstrated that as a group, nurses who work predominantly at night are disadvantaged in many ways and for a variety of reasons. Whilst nurse managers and the profession as a whole have a responsibility to address some of the issues, the best people to tackle most of these problems are the nurses themselves. Only by becoming proactive both in care and politically will they be able to achieve change in their situation. This means demonstrating knowledge, ability and enthusiasm for care; it means becoming assertive and expressing how the nurse feels to colleagues and managers, and it means being creative to solve clinical and managerial problems in a way that benefits patients whilst at the same time contributing to the achievement of organisational objectives.

The future of nursing at night is in the balance; it is up to nurses who work at that time to take the lead in making it an effective and respected service.

References

Adam K (1980) Dietary habits and sleep after bedtime food drinks. *Sleep*, **3**, 1, 47–58.

Armstrong M (1987) No proper time of day. *Occupational Health*, **39**, 2, 54–56.

Aurell J and Elmqvist D (1985) Sleep in the surgical intensive care unit: continuous polygraphic recording of sleep in nine patients receiving postoperative care. *British Medical Journal*, **290**, 1029–1032.

Brezinova V and Oswald I (1972) Sleep after a bedtime beverage. *British Medical Journal*, **2**, 5811, 431–433.

Canavan T (1986) The functions of sleep. *Nursing*, **3**, 9, 321–324.

Carskadon M A, Dement W C, Mitler M M, Guilleminault C, Zarcone V P and Spiegel R (1976) Self-reports versus sleep laboratory findings in 122 drug-free subjects with complaints of chronic insomnia. *American Journal of Psychiatry*, **133**, 1382–1388.

Closs S J (1988) *A Nursing Study of Sleep on Surgical Wards*. University of Edinburgh Department of Nursing Studies.

Darragh A, Lambe R F, Hallinhan D and O'Kelly M M (1979) Caffeine in soft drinks. *Lancet*, **1**, 1196.

Ersser S (1991) A search for the therapeutic dimensions of nurse-patient interaction. In McMahon R and Pearson A (eds) *Nursing as Therapy*. London: Chapman and Hall.

Evers H K (1981a) Care or custody? The experience of women patients in long stay geriatric wards. In Hutter B and Williams G (eds) *Controlling Women: The Normal and the Deviant*. London: Croom Helm.

Evers H K (1981b) Tender loving care? Nurses and patients in geriatric wards. In Copp L A (ed) *Recent Advances in Nursing 2: Care of the Ageing*. Edinburgh: Churchill Livingstone.

Glover M (1986) Drugs for poor sleepers? *British Medical Journal*, **292**, 1200.

Gournay K (1988) Sleeping without drugs. *Nursing Times*, **84**, 11, 46–49.

Halfens R, Lendfers M L and Cox K (1988) Nurse characteristics and their effect on sleep medication. *Nursing Times*, **84**, 43, 74.

Hamric A B and Spross J A (1989) *The Clinical Nurse Specialist in Theory and Practice (2nd Edition)*. Philadelphia: W B Saunders Co.

Karacan I, Thornby J I, Anch A M, Booth G H, Williams R L and Salis P J (1976) Dose-related sleep disturbances induced by coffee and caffeine. *Clin. Pharmacol. Ther.*, **20**, 682–689.

Levy M and Zylber-Katz E (1983) Caffeine metabolism and coffee attributed sleep disturbances. *Clin. Pharmacol. Ther.*, **33**, 770–775.

Lloyd P (1989) Nurses working at night-time: the forgotten army. *Lampada* , **1**, 19, 13–14.

McMahon R (1990) Sleep management. *Surgical Nurse*, **3**, 4, 25–27.

McMahon R (1991) Therapeutic nursing: theory, issues and practice. In McMahon R and Pearson A (eds) *Nursing as Therapy*. London: Chapman and Hall.

Minors D, Waterhouse J and Folkard S (1985) When duty calls. *Nursing Times*, November 13th, 27–28.

Morgan K (1987) *Sleep and Ageing*. London: Croom Helm.

Morgan K, Healey D W and Healey P J (1989) Factors influencing persistent subjective insomnia in old age: a follow-up study of good and poor sleepers aged 65 to 74. *Age and Aging*, **18**, 117–122.

NHS Management Consultancy Services (1987) *Study of Night Nursing Services*. London: DHSS.

Ogilvie A J (1980) Sources and levels of noise on the ward at night. *Nursing Times*, July 31st, 1363–1366.

Oswald I (1986) Drugs for poor sleepers? *British Medical Journal*, **292**, 715.

Paterson J G and Zderad L T (1976) *Humanistic Nursing*. New York: John Wiley.

Pawlicki R E (1985) Behavioural management of insomnia. *Psychosocial Nursing*, **23**, 7, 14–17.

Post-registration Education and Practice Project (1990) *Report of the Post-Registration Education and Practice Project*. London: UKCC.

Rundell O H, Lester B K, Griffiths W J and Williams H L (1972) Alcohol and sleep in young adults. *Psychopharmacologia*, **26**, 201–218.

Smith M (1990) Making the most of the CNS. *Senior Nurse*, **10**, 9, 6–8.

Soldatos C R, Kales J D, Scharf M B, Bixle E O and Kales A (1980) Cigarette smoking associated with sleep difficulty. *Science*, **207**, 551–553.

Torrance C (1990) Sleep and wound healing. *Surgical Nurse*, **3**, 3, 17–22.

Weiss B L et al (1973) Once more, the inaccuracy of non-EEG estimates of sleep. *American Journal of Psychiatry*, **130**, 1282–1285.

Wright S (1989) *Changing Nursing Practice*. London: Edward Arnold.

Index